THE

CURE

A Novel by:
Robert K. Oldham, M.D.

First printing, 1991

PUBLISHED BY PULSE PUBLICATIONS, INC.
Franklin, TN 37065

Library of Congress Catalog Card No: 90-92322
ISBN: 0-9628850-0-2

Printed in the United States of America

DEDICATION AND ACKNOWLEDGEMENTS

This book is dedicated to my patients past, present and future. They truly understand the search for *THE CURE.*

My heartfelt thanks to my wife Cathie, my children Robert II, Andrew, Clarke, Daniel and Bo for their support and to the staff of BTI and PPI for their assistance.

Special thanks are due J. Anthony Forstmann. Without Mr. Forstmann's support it would have been impossible to develop BTI.

THE CURE was published through financial assistance and general support of Cathie's father and mother, James R. and Miriam H. Moon.

Robert K. Oldham, M.D.
January 4, 1991

PREFACE

Cancer is a devastating disease. Even for the cured, the treatments are harsh and side effects debilitating. Americans believe in technology. They believe that technology will bring cures for many diseases. Specifically, the search for the cure for cancer has been a persistent dream of patients and scientists.

Cancer research is envisioned as good. The people and institutions involved in cancer research are generally considered to be working in the public's interest with the patient's needs as the primary motivation.

This novel describes the plight of five cancer patients who use their resources in an attempt to find the cure for their soon-to-be lethal cancer. The characters are all fictional but representative of many cancer patients who actively search for improved treatment for their disease. The frustration of the search and difficulty in understanding the cancer research maze is outlined by each patient's search for the cure. Persistence, money, power, political intrigue and even the telephone are all resources to them. Each frantically tries to understand and utilize the cancer research and treatment system before it is too late.

Four major characters, all physicians, illustrate the inner workings of the cancer research and treatment system that the patients are attempting to understand and utilize. Also fictional, these individuals represent composite personalities from government, university and the private sector in a patchwork system of cancer care.

Through the development of these characters, the interactions between the patient and the complex system are revealed.

Panic, despair, ecstasy, success and failure, as well as power, greed, money and commitment are the driving forces of the individuals caught in the web of these interactions. Through the lives of the patients and physicians, this novel gives a truly insightful view of America's healthcare system, its successes and its failures.

OVERVIEW

CHAPTER 1 "Portrait of a Cancer Patient" (3/1/84)

The story opens in 1984 with a not well-to-do, unsophisticated Georgia shop owner, Lydia Green, about to receive further chemotherapy for her lymphoma. She is sick, uncomfortable and in the hospital with drug resistant lymphoma. The story opens with her questioning Dr. Gordon about why she has to receive more chemotherapy; whether it might be better to just die. At the same time, she asks a hundred questions about biological treatments and whether they might be more effective and less toxic. Her distress is extreme, her questions pertinent, and the issues unresolvable. This dilemma of the sick patient confronting the physician with unanswerable questions and the secondary dilemma of Dr. Gordon knowing that there are potential new approaches for the patient which he is unable to provide because of limited access to new technologies will be apparent. Much of the first chapter revolves around Lydia Green's physical pain and the physician's emotional pain and discomfort in being unable to pursue suitable research options because of the "system." These issues and their discussion through this patient's case sets the stage for the whole novel demonstrating barriers in the search for the cure.

As will be the case throughout "THE CURE", the individual characters will be used to discuss generic problems and to emphasize and highlight, through their personal experiences, the system restrictions in bringing to bear available resources in cancer research and treatment to the benefit of patients.

CHAPTER 2 "Rise to the Top" (1/79)

This chapter develops the character of Stephen Musso. It begins by going back in time to his youth and describes his growth and development as a student, physician and later a major figure within the Federal Cancer Institute (FCI). It describes his character and demonstrates his motivations and modus operandi. It begins in the 1940s and 1950s and ends in the mid-1970s with the development of effective chemotherapy for lymphoma, a project where he is perceived to have played the major role. The chapter ends with Stephen aspiring to be Director of the FCI, by ruthlessly consolidating his power at the expense of others. His thoughts and plans to achieve his personal goals and expand his powerbase through the use of political forces and the creation of a "family," will illustrate the way personal interests and power seeking drive the FCI system.

CHAPTER 3 Top Dog" (Fall 1979)

By Fall 1979, Stephen Musso's plans are complete. After meticulous preparation, he is prepared to make his final strategic move, to replace Jacob Poldosky as Director, FCI. Manipulating people is Stephen's specialty. Now, one last manipulation to take him to the top.

CHAPTER 4 "Fall From Grace" (Summer 1980)

Daniel C. Weil's background and development in becoming the Chairman of the Board of a large chemical company is described. Mr. Weil is relatively old when he uses the system for his benefit after a long and productive life as an industrialist in the chemical industry. The chapter demonstrates his insensitivity to society's exposure to potential carcinogenic chemical compounds handled by his company. He is clearly identified as an individual both interested in personal gain and relatively ruthless with respect to his business practices. He uses his power to do what he wants to the exclusion of others. A dedicated family man, Daniel is a great patriarch of his company and family; a great patriot of the system. He will be in his late 70's in 1980, diagnosed as having lung cancer and begins his search for "the cure." It begins at the pinnacle of his power and ends with him in the hospital contemplating his mortality.

CHAPTER 5 "The Commitment" (1959 - 1963)

Dr. Robert Gordon's character is developed from early childhood through medical school and residency training. This chapter explores, through his eyes, the sense of frustration on the part of both the patient and physician in these attempts to use current and future technology for the benefit of the patient. It ends with him anticipating being able to do much more for patients by virtue of the upcoming FCI training period.

This chapter states the problem and outlines the conflicts and difficulties in cancer research focusing on the developing feelings of a young physician dedicated to cancer patients. It conveys Robert's belief that better training will allow him to do all the things he wants to do for patients. This is based on the belief that the research system is available to serve all patients once the physician acquires a more complete understanding. His belief in the purity of science, the dedication of medical researchers, and the opportunities available allow the reader to sense the measure of a young physician going forth to acquire the tools to conquer the problem of cancer.

CHAPTER 6 "The Task Force" (6/80)

This chapter traces a powerful oil man, John J. Owens, from his ascension to power within the Texas petroleum industry to his diagnosis of colon cancer. His organization of an effort to solve his problem and find the best treatment for his colon cancer focuses on the character but will examine certain aspects of the university system within the United States as this wealthy individual looks at ways to use various university programs for personal benefit. It describes his early attempts to influence the system on his behalf as he proposes gifts and grants, in the philanthropic mode, with the unstated presumption that university and government researchers will work diligently to solve his personal problem. The institutions suggest laboratories and buildings be named for him but do not respond in the way he desires, i.e. finding a specific treatment for his specific cancer. This chapter ends with John J. continuing his search for "the cure" through treatment at the FCI.

CHAPTER 7 "Nobel Ambitions" (8/79)

The chapter opens with an argument between Dr. Salla and Dr. George Trumpey, a competitive researcher, with the focus on a "laboratory accident" and the discovery of a new virus. It uses flashbacks to describe Dr. Salla's earlier development, his relationship with Stephen and allows the reader to understand the powerful position that Dr. Salla has within the FCI in the early 1980s. It describes processes in the laboratory used to isolate viruses and the many manipulations that take place to obtain specimens, money, research laboratory space, technical slots, etc. from the government research establishment through personal influence, bribery, manipulation, and scientific accomplishment in the search for "the cure." Dr. Salla's shark-like character illustrates his unending thrust for power and the Nobel Prize.

CHAPTER 8 "The Shattered Dream" (Fall 1956)

Senator Robert Tomasi's character, his shining image as a rising star in politics is briefly outlined; an individual unsullied by the political process, a man well educated and thoughtful about human interactions and a person dedicated to being forthright and direct, who is attempting to maintain his personal integrity by not using the political system to which he is so well attuned. His personal gregariousness and political popularity prompts his grooming by family and friends to become President of the United States. His dedication to correcting the inequities of the political system are folded into the story line. Thus, through this chapter one sees the aspiring optimist, an image the Senator has for himself and one the well polished candidate carefully constructs with his family and his political constituency to achieve the goal of becoming President. The presidency would allow him to pursue innermost desires to correct certain aspects of the system and to reduce the political patronage that he sees as so great a problem.

In the context of these very strong feelings, the Senator develops lymphoma. This diagnosis becomes a major logistical, emotional, and intellectual problem for him. Someone ill with lymphoma cannot become President, so he must find "the cure." It is emotional in that it destroys his dreams of fixing the system by becoming the leader. It is an intellectual dilemma by virtue of the understanding he has of the political system and how it can be used to help him personally, knowledge that is the antithesis of his inner desires. He has the obvious dilemma of whether to be true to his inner feelings or whether to use the system to his own benefit in an attempt to find a cure. He sees the obvious dichotomy in that he can use the system, perhaps find a cure, achieve the position of leader, go back and perhaps change the system.

CHAPTER 9 "Telephone Research" (Fall 1975)

Sam Luria, the Greek Restauranteur, is a persistent, probing man with the ability to hold the listener's attention on the telephone to extract information. Sam is the best informed myeloma patient in the world and he is the world's best at using the telephone to gather information and take action. He doesn't have the resources of a rich man but like Lydia Green, he uses his own resources in the search for "the cure."

CHAPTER 10 "Using the System" (1968)

This chapter concerns The Lizard, Dr. Stanley Lizzard, and gives a very brief biographical sketch of this individual. His growth in a Jewish ghetto in Newark, New Jersey, the clawing to the top through attachments to various individuals, especially Stephen, and his reward in the appointment to become the Cancer Therapy Division Director as Stephen ascends to the Directorship of the FCI. The dialogue very sharply focuses on The Lizard and his role as Stephen's henchman. Like Stephen, Stanley is associated with the development of drugs for cancer treatment and will have a strong political and scientific allegiance to this area. He is characterized by his ability to shake hands, pat people on the back, reward and punish; all in a rather slimy way. On the surface, he is always described as a leader in drug metabolism and scientific thought but under the surface, many recognize him for what he is, a mean-spirited character, who has risen to a position of power primarily through his relationship to Stephen Musso.

CHAPTER 11 "Back to the University" (7/5/70)

Robert Gordon completes his research at the FCI and faces the dilemma of whether to stay in the federal system or return to the university. After a great deal of debate, he elects to return to the university thinking he will have more flexibility and opportunity.

The move to Mallory University represents a return to the south for Mary Margaret, Robert's wife. She and the family are very pleased to be back "home." Robert begins his work in Atlanta with a great deal of fundraising and patient care activity hoping to develop the laboratory capabilities needed to support a major program in research. Genetic engineering and hybridoma technology have just come on the scene. Robert sees the opportunities for major advances in cancer research to the benefit of his patients, but lacks the revenues and power to pursue them.

CHAPTER 12 "Prizes Large and Small" (1980)

Chapter 10 and 11 will highlight the recent biological "revolution." Through remarkable advances in biology, molecular biology, computer· technology and hybridoma technology events come together in the late 1980's to give a basis for a new thought process in cancer biology such that biological materials might be used to better understand cancer and might be used directly in cancer treatment. The biological revolution of the 1970's brings biotherapy to the fore as a potential fourth treatment modality to be added to surgery, radiation and chemotherapy. Chapter 12 outlines some of the hypocrisy of university medicine demonstrating how academia tends to restrict information to itself unless publication of the information serves to aggrandize the individual. It highlights certain aspects of prizes and rewards within the academic system and will demonstrate how more and more prizes and awards such as the Wilson Medal are coming forth to publicly reward scientists for their achievements. There is a mixture of good and dedicated integrated with the egotistical and power seeking intrinsic to the cancer research establishment, the "system."

CHAPTER 13 "The FCI Biotherapy Program and the Test Pilot" (February 1980)

Through Chapter 12, the stage has been set for the development of a major program in "new biology" within the FCI. The players are in place, the biological revolution has occurred, Dr. Gordon's character and career have matured. It opens after Stephen Musso's ascension to the Directorship of the FCI and his decision that a biotherapy program will need sufficient resources to develop but not so many resources to develop too quickly. He agrees to find a person for the program who can be used and then eliminated, if necessary, because they may need to put one of their own inner circle in the leadership position. They mandate a trial period of two to three years and then to set up a "review" scenario; if the program needs to be reorganized in the usual FCI fashion, by using criticism and outside peer review to demonstrate the lack of ability or success for the current program and its director, they can reorganize it into a "new" program. By removing the initial program director, Stephen can take credit for its success and tailor it to his own future needs. Dr. Robert Gordon is much discussed with respect to risks and rewards in asking him to direct the program. Against Stanley Lizzard's instincts, Stephen decides, with FCI Executive Committee concurrence, to offer Robert the Directorship.

CHAPTER 14 "The Decision" (Fall 1980)

Dr. Gordon must consider another major decision. His aspirations for the development of cancer biotherapy are apparent and his thoughts and frustrations about not being able to achieve sufficient critical laboratory mass are the critical factors. His five years at Mallory demonstrated his leadership capabilities in the area of medical oncology and documented his abilities as an immunologist and scientist as well as a clinician. By 1980, he is considered a young leader in the area of medical oncology, a medical oncologist who is somewhat of an individualist. He will be seen as an individual who speaks his mind, is unafraid of criticizing the university system, as well as an individual who is somewhat controversial by virtue of his directness and outspoken approach. In spite of all these "bad qualities," Dr. Gordon is admired and respected for his honesty, integrity and dedication to delivering new treatments for patients.

It is Fall 1980, when out of the blue an offer comes from the FCI to lead their new program in biotherapy. This offer brings major controversy to his life. He must resolve his professional needs with his personal responsibilities. After much soul-searching and discussion with his family (but not with the university), he abruptly decides to take the job and notifies Mallory. This decision, which he attempts to present in a "leave of absence" arrangement which might strengthen the university in the future, is not met with general approval. The chapter ends with his acceptance of the appointment to head the FCI Biotherapy Program.

CHAPTER 15 "Contacts" (July 1982)

Chapter 15 opens with Dr. Gordon's arrival at the FCI. This segment follows the development of the program, recruitment of scientists, openings of laboratories, and the beginning of a world class research program in biotherapy. Much of the logistical development and political battles in initiating the program will be described.

Some of the patients now come back into play. The Connecticut industrialist makes his initial contact to the FCI through Dr. Salla. The Senator makes his contact through Stephen and the Texas oil man through his Senator. This chapter describes the scientific progress of biotherapy in the FCI over approximately a two year period. Some of these patients are brought into focus in their search for the cure. The biotherapy program and Dr. Gordon illustrate interactions that can occur in trying to use the government and university system for the benefit of individual patients.

CHAPTER 16 "Success Means Failure" (September 1982)

Success is apparent for the Biotherapy Program with worldwide recognition, and the continued political battles within the FCI. A secret meeting of Stephen Musso and his henchmen occurs and the decision will be made to replace Dr. Gordon as Director. He is becoming too vocal, too public and too successful taking away from the attention that Stephen would prefer to come through Dr. Salla, the Lizard, Dr. Brody and himself for the FCI in Washington so he might be glorified by his initiatives. The decision is made to make times difficult for Dr. Gordon with the intent of replacing him as soon as possible.

CHAPTER 17 "The Break" (September 1983)

Stephen Musso makes a promise and a threat. The promise is that if Dr. Gordon will remain quiet, then Stephen will give him strong, positive recommendations and support saying that he left under the best of circumstances with the full support of the FCI; contrary to this, if Dr. Gordon elects to "go public" the recommendation will be negative, the press will be bad, and it will be publicly stated that he was asked to leave the FCI. This represents a challenge since Dr. Gordon can see that a negative recommendation may lead to difficulty developing a private initiative. He faces a similar dilemma as Senator Tomasi in asking himself if he should defer his long term aspirations and integrity to get past the short term problem so he might be ultimately successful in changing the system.

CHAPTER 18 "Cancer Therapeutics Inc." (January 1984)

Robert Gordon writes a business plan setting out to begin a private enterprise company to deliver biotherapy to patients. This chapter will go through the financial steps necessary to establish the company. Some of the presentations, the acquisition of early individuals to carry out the work of the company, and a description of what goes on in establishing this new company called Cancer Therapeutics Inc. (CTI) are included. Richard Toban, Bill Carothers and the private investors commit and CTI is funded, certain scientists are brought on board, and the aspirations of its founder, Dr. Gordon, are clearly outlined. Business is business and science is science, but the two come together for CTI.

CHAPTER 19 "The Headline was Dramatic" (Fall 1984)

The FCI announces the long sought after viral cause of lymphoma by describing HLV-1 in Journal of Science and in the press. This discovery, which has major scientific implications, is lost on Lydia Green who has the practical problem of what to do about her lymphoma. Dr. Gordon asked Lydia if she would like to participate as a research patient in the CTI anti-idiotypic antibody program. This requires a lymph node to be delivered to the laboratory for an attempt at making antibodies specific for Lydia's tumor. This approach represents the culmination of Lydia's dream that a biological based treatment might someday be developed and be useful in her particular situation. She readily agrees to proceed with this approach and feels a great sense of satisfaction over finally having the opportunity to participate in this type of research.

CHAPTER 20 "The Case" (Spring 1985)

Daniel Weil is treated with interferon but denied access to IL-2 activated cells. Stanley Lizzard discharges him summarily. Mr. Weil is not a good candidate for experimental treatment. He goes to Dr. Gordon for options.

CHAPTER 21 "Cocktails for Cancer" (Summer 1985)

John J. Owens, the most researched, single human cancer patient ever, decides to see Dr. Gordon. His research team recommends that the monoclonal antibody cocktail approach is best and that John J. should proceed in seeing Dr. Gordon and supporting his novel approach.

CHAPTER 22 "Suspicion" (Spring 1985)

The 1985 Wilson Prize goes to Dr. Stephen Musso. On the surface, all is well, but Stephen is worried. There are some undercurrents to indicate that major problems may be brewing at the FCI. Two new names arise -- Martin Bartholomew and Constance Kelley. No real connection but two "problems" arising at the same time. Stephen's antennas are up.

CHAPTER 23 "Private Research" (Fall 1985)

Senator Tomasi resolves his "ethical" concerns and decides to go for monoclonal antibody therapy in Atlanta. He has hedged his bets with a variety of institutions and now wants a private sector approach to further open his options for future treatment.

CHAPTER 24 "Rounds" (Spring 1986)

Good Samaritan Hospital has taken on the CTI Program and becomes a center of national attention for private-sector cancer research. Mr. Weil, Ms. Green, Mr. Owens and Sam Luria are all seen on rounds, some under treatment, some not, but all with a great deal of enthusiasm for the CTI mission.

CHAPTER 25 "Warheads and Cocktails" (Summer 1986)

The laboratory report and the mouse studies on Senator Tomasi are highly encouraging. At last, evidence that an antibody cocktail properly linked to multiple drugs, could have significant effects on cancer growth. The CTI antibody "multiple warhead" immunoconjugate approach is ready for the clinic. The Senator is to be the first human ever treated with this new approach. If successful, Senator Tomasi will be ready to run for the Presidency.

CHAPTER 26 "Full Circle" (Fall 1986)

The drug development program at FCI comes under scrutiny because of huge expenditures and little progress over two decades. A reporter's "insider information" and a series of articles in the Washington Post spell major trouble for Stephen Musso and his FCI family. New winds were blowing in the federal program. It is time for a new leader.

CHAPTER 27 "The Prize" (1987)

Roger Salla wins the 1987 Nobel Prize for medicine based on his discovery of a virus which causes colon cancer. This discovery and the prize validates the "big science" approach of the FCI. Individuals come and go but the system persists and prospers.

EPILOGUE

Mr. Weil, Mr. Owens, Mr. Luria and Ms. Green have their medical status reviewed. Senator Tomasi, Drs. Salla and Musso move on to bigger and better things. Stanley Lizzard dies. His work unfinished, Robert Gordon continues to develop the CTI paradigm.

CHAPTER 1

PORTRAIT OF A CANCER PATIENT

March 1, 1984

The warmth on her eyelids told Lydia Green that she had survived another night. And the tightness in her chest meant that she had awakened to another day with cancer.

How long had it been now? Ten years since she had found the first lump, a tiny bit of probably nothing in her throat.

"Don't worry, it's probably nothing," that's what Dr. Fremont, the first in a long line of doctors, had said. But he'd wanted to do a biopsy anyway, to rule out Hodgkin's disease, he'd said, smiling as he told her not to worry, in that way that doctors had of hiding the truth for as long as they could get away with it. He, the nurse, and the secretary had been almost obnoxiously cheery as they set up an appointment for the biopsy.

But Lydia had instinctively known that something was wrong.

Shortly before the appointment for the biopsy, she ducked into the library at the medical center. She had felt a little out of place amongst the always-in-a-hurry doctors and medical students, but had summoned up the courage to ask the librarian to help her find some books on Hodgkin's disease. The librarian had actually seemed a little relieved to be helping a normal, non-medical person.

Lydia had heard of people getting Hodgkin's, but thought that they were usually young, not in their late forties like her. She was shocked to learn that Hodgkin's disease was a deadly cancer. And one that she might have. Why hadn't Dr. Fremont told her more? Probably because he hadn't wanted her to worry. Suddenly the lump in her throat seemed the size of a grapefruit.

The biopsy itself was unpleasant, but not as dreadful as Lydia had imagined. Her real distress came after the procedure, when she lay in the cold, dreary recovery room awaiting the results. She was wheeled in, parked in a corner and ignored, left for an endless hour to wonder whether or not she had a terminal illness. And just when she was beginning to think that they had mistaken her for a corpse and would soon move her to a medical school dissection class, Dr. Fremont came in. She was shivering, too petrified to ask the obvious question, and the fact that the doctor had his face buried in her chart alarmed her further. But the news, she had thought, was actually good -- it wasn't Hodgkin's after all. And that was all Lydia had heard. If it wasn't Hodgkin's, then it must be benign. Now, though, she could dimly recall the rest of his sentence -- "but it's a non- Hodgkin's form of lymphoma."

Dr. Fremont had either neglected to tell her -- or confused and isolated, she had neglected to hear -- that her lymphoma was a disease for which there was no cure. It, too, was cancer, and she had it.

But at the time, all she could feel was overwhelming relief that it wasn't the dreaded Hodgkin's disease. Now all they had done was take out the lump, and she could forget about it. She'd never have to see the grinning Dr. Fremont again. She could get on with her life.

Later, she was a little surprised when the doctor wanted to examine her more closely and take some x-rays, to help him treat her problem. Of course, she had understood. As long as the thing growing in her throat wasn't Hodgkins.

So she had been poked and prodded, then x-rayed, and sent home.

The next week, she went again to Dr. Fremont's office. The cheshire-cat secretary and nurse were as falsely cheerful as ever, but it didn't really bother her this time, because she knew she wouldn't be coming here long. But she was wrong. The x-rays had shown a lump growing near her stomach similar to the one removed from her throat. It could be unrelated, Dr. Fremont had said, but he really didn't think so. She'd need some treatment. He didn't want to take any chances.

Lydia refused to become alarmed. She had heard his words but surely he must have made a mistake, probably confused her tests with some other poor soul's. After all, she didn't have any stomach pain, so how could there be a lump there? And what did he mean by 'take any chances'?"

Dr. Fremont had then patiently explained that the two lumps -- the one in her throat and the one that she couldn't feel but was nonetheless growing near her stomach -- were most likely part of the same disease process, part of her non-Hodgkin's lymphoma. She had certainly been relieved to hear the "non-Hodgkin's" part. What the doctor planned to do was to treat Lydia's whole system to make sure every bit of the lymphoma would shrink and disappear, rather than cutting it out piece by piece. In other words, drugs and radiation would be used instead of surgery. That was fine with Lydia. It seemed to make sense, and didn't sound too painful or expensive.

And so the cobalt treatments had begun, along with her first chemotherapy, in tablet form. She'd been a little nauseous, but it wasn't really too bad. And five months after she had started on the combined treatment, Dr. Fremont told her that x-rays had shown that the lymphoma had stopped growing. Patient and doctor were delighted.

Lydia had enjoyed four "disease-free" years that first time. She had thought that she had seen the last of the evil lumps, that she was cured. But all that was long ago. Today, March 1, 1984, was an anniversary of sorts. For that first lymphoma had been found exactly a decade ago.

"Good morning, Ms. Green. Did you sleep well? Time for our morning blood work."

The annoying singsong voice of nurse Copeland brought Lydia back to the present, a not unpleasant semi-private room in Good Samaritan Hospital, ten miles from her home in Fairfield, Georgia. Lydia intensely disliked nurse Copeland. If it's "our" blood, I wish she could take some of my needle sticks, Lydia thought bitterly. But she somehow managed to answer semi-civilly, "My back doesn't seem to be too bad yet, but I can think of a nicer way to get up than being stabbed again. Which arm this time?" she said as she offered both. Lydia barely even felt the needles anymore.

"The left will do fine," nurse Copeland answered. "You're in luck. In a little while Dr. Gordon will be making his rounds," offered the nurse as she capped the vacutainer needle. "You can bombard him with questions then," she added, glancing over to the pile of books on the night table. Lydia smiled. She knew that "a little while" in a hospital could mean half the morning, or even longer. So she settled back into the pillows to get more sleep before the nurse with the medicine tray came rattling around. But she was uncomfortable and was anxious about meeting the eminent Dr. Gordon. Now that she was so close to finally talking to him, she was uncharacteristically nervous, and hoped that she could remember to ask all of the questions that she had been carefully compiling.

Lydia had had to apply to participate in Dr. Gordon's experimental clinical trials. She had been chosen from many patients because of her strength, stamina, and good health, besides the cancer, of course. At this first meeting, she and the doctor were to talk about yet another new drug regimen. This would be her fourth -- or was it her fifth? -- type of chemotherapy. She didn't really want to do it though. She'd certainly had her fill of chemicals, but her daughter had persuaded her to give conventional treatment another try, after reading a newspaper account that made Dr. Gordon seem a little different from the rest. But Lydia knew deep down that this chemotherapy would fail. They all did.

She remembered how devastated she had been the first time the tumors had returned.

It had been four years after her initial cobalt and chemotherapy sessions -- four fairly normal years during which she had seen her two daughters reach adulthood and launched her handicrafts shop, "Miscellaneous". This time it wasn't her throat or her stomach that sent her back to Dr. Fremont, but her lungs, which had filled painfully with fluid. She thought it was pneumonia, not the cancer. But Dr. Fremont became alarmed, although of course he tried to hide it. He said it was due to the lymphoma.

Lydia was utterly confused and terrified because she had been certain that the cancer was gone. (By this time she had finally figured out that non-Hodgkin's lymphoma was indeed cancer.) And now it was much more painful. She had the fluid drained from her lungs, which offered some relief, albeit temporary. A large needle pushed into her chest like a knife stab in an alley, 20 times that year. And she began another round of chemotherapy.

At first, Lydia didn't understand why she'd have to take more drugs. If chemotherapy hadn't worked the first time, what made the doctor think it would work now? Dr. Fremont explained that she'd be getting a different combination of drugs that kills cancer cells in a different way from the first drug regimen. Also, cancer cells change, and the ones in her lungs may not be at all like those in her throat and stomach.

Lydia hadn't understood what that meant either, and again she asked him why he thought another go at "chemo" would work. And she was surprised when he admitted that he really didn't know whether it would work or not, that he was just trying different approaches, hoping it wouldn't be long before they found something that proved effective. She was both happy that he was finally being honest with her and alarmed by his admitted uncertainty. Doctors weren't supposed to have doubts. This cancer treatment business was beginning to seem almost like a lottery, she had said, and again, he had agreed. He told her that each time the cancer returned, it could be more resistant to particular drugs, and new ones would have to be sought. But fortunately, it turned out that there was quite an arsenal of chemotherapies for lymphoma. Dr. Fremont had actually called her "lucky" in having her particular type of cancer, because it was slow- growing and responsive to many drugs. Easy for him to say. He didn't feel like there was a knife in his chest every time he breathed.

But Lydia's drug treatment this time around wasn't quite as simple. Just a few hours after returning home from her visit to the doctor, Lydia began throwing up, and continued to vomit for the next 24 hours. The nausea was relentless, overpowering and terrifying. And two weeks after the therapy had begun, she awoke one morning to find most of her beautiful, dark blond hair fanned out on the pillow. Just passing a comb through her hair finished the job. She cried for two days and couldn't leave the house for a week. The chemotherapy was obviously harming more than just the cancer cells. And was it really doing any good?

The noisy entry of the day nurse wheeling in the medicine tray brought Lydia back to the present.

"Good morning Ms. Green," chirped the nurse. This was a new one, probably straight out of school, from the looks of her. "Pill time." Silently Lydia swallowed the antibiotic tablets. What would happen, she often wondered, if she refused to take them, and let nature take its course? According to the doctors, she'd get a whopping infection. Immune suppression and all that. But she was beginning not to care.

"Good girl," cooed the nurse. This one must had been trained in pediatrics, Lydia thought. She knew what would come next. "Now it's time for our vitamins."

What a joke. Vitamins and minerals. "I've had enough vitamins and minerals to last many lifetimes," Lydia grumbled. Her quest for alternative cancer treatments had included pounds of vitamins. She had begun her search in 1980, after her devastating experience with chemotherapy.

It had gotten to the point that she just couldn't take it anymore. Her dread of receiving chemotherapy was by now almost as bad as the agony of the treatment itself. Poisoning the body didn't seem a logical way to restore health to it. And so she had begged Dr. Fremont to find a treatment that wouldn't make her more sick than the illness it was supposed to cure.

The doctor had seemed a bit uncomfortable, as if he'd run into this problem before. He launched into his usual speech about her "disseminated lymphoma", and how they should continue experimenting with new drugs, draining her lungs to relieve her pain, and pumping her full of antibiotics to discourage infection. She could practically make the speech herself.

He wasn't relieving her pain, he was only substituting it with another, worse kind, she thought. There just had to be a more natural way to fight this thing. After all, the cancer had arisen naturally, because she didn't smoke or drink alcohol or coffee or do drugs or lie in the sun or work with toxic chemicals or eat hot dogs or other processed foods or anything else that's supposed to cause cancer. She was thin, active, with a happy life. She'd done nothing to deserve this. It was only logical that if the cancer had arisen naturally, it could be beaten naturally.

The doctor hadn't answered immediately. Finally, he admitted that he understood how she felt (but how could he?), and that if it would make her feel better, then she should seek alternative treatments. But he cautioned her that she'd probably end up back with him, or with another doctor who'd also recommend chemotherapy. He had looked defeated, and for the first time, Lydia actually felt sorry for him.

So Lydia had been set free to roam to book stores and library shelves, in search of a more "natural" cancer treatment. She tried everything. Megavitamins and macrobiotics, mineral supplements, kelp, raw vegetables, water therapy, vitamin C injections. She went to doctors of varying capabilities in five stages, spending a month here, a week there, having her lungs drained occasionally. She tried DMSO in Oregon and laetrile in Mexico. She tried other doctors and other drugs, whatever she heard of. She could have supplied "60 Minutes" with stories of cancer quackery for a year. She tried coffee enemas and mental imaging, mind- over-matter to will the destruction of her cancerous cells. There were urine extract injections from a zoologist in Bermuda, and a visit to an Arizona clinic that promised "tumorex and other support modalities, including DMSO, live cell therapy, Gerovital, enzyme therapy, cardiovascular chelation, nutritional education, colonic irrigation, reflexology, irridiology, and deep nerve, deep tissue, lymphatic and shiatzu massage therapies." This place had sounded great, until the Food and Drug Administration (FDA) shut it down.

After three years of search for magic, Lydia had returned to Georgia and Dr. Fremont, her bowels and purse cleansed, her ying and yang in perfect balance, probably better nourished, but exhausted both from her traveling and from her relentless disease. And she presented the doctor with a rather impossible situation -- she wanted him to drain her lungs periodically, but to think of some way other than drugs to treat the cancer.

But it just couldn't be done. And she would never forget what the doctor had said next. "Lydia, I don't know what the hell I'm going to do with you now. You've tried all of those crazy treatments and now you want me to treat you without using chemotherapy." Case closed. He had officially given up. Annoyed with the doctor's callousness, but not too surprised, Lydia left. She'd just take it day by day, and see how she could function without his medical help.

Each day was different. Some days she managed to get to her handicrafts shop, now run by one of her daughters. If she sat doing billing or making phone calls, she could make it through the day. Other mornings she'd awaken, take a brisk shower, eat breakfast, and then collapse in bed and stay there all day, totally exhausted. She lost many days to colds and sore throats. And there were days when she could barely breathe because of the fluid in her lungs and the pain on inhaling because of the tumors in her back. When she took a deep breath, the pain was like a searing hot metal probe slicing through her flesh. She had learned to breathe as shallowly as possible, but every once in a while she'd forget herself and inhale deeply, which temporarily incapacitated her. She knew that the pain couldn't be tolerated much longer.

A sunny Tuesday in the winter of 1984 had been a turning point -- or at least she had hoped it would be. Her daughter had found her in bed at 8 a.m., in too much pain to even cry out. She couldn't even sit up. Her always efficient elder daughter had quickly taken charge, making her mother more comfortable, and calling her sister to watch the store. Then she had stepped outside to pick up the newspaper from the porch.

A few minutes later she had rushed back in, obviously excited, scanning an article on the front page. A new cancer specialist was planning to open a "revolutionary new" treatment facility right there in Fairfield.

Lydia hadn't wanted to squelch her daughter's hopes, but she was so sick of the cancer treatment merry-go-round that she just couldn't keep her thoughts to herself. "Another drug pusher, that's all," she whined.

No wonder Dee hadn't refused to give up. You never knew, she'd said many times, when the right drug would come along, and you certainly wouldn't know if you didn't try. Dee had urged Lydia to at least see the new doctor. And if she refused, she'd drag her there.

As her daughter read on, she became even more excited. It seemed that Dr. Gordon was going to try a whole new approach to cancer treatment. But Lydia was still skeptical. Just a new name for the same old thing. What could it be, if not chemotherapy, radiation or surgery? Dee starting reading aloud:

> *"Dr. Gordon comes back to his Georgia roots from the Federal Cancer Institute, where he headed the Cancer Biotherapy Program for nearly four years. An expert in chemotherapy, Dr. Gordon is also at the forefront of cancer research, exploring the body's own cancer-fighting chemicals, called biological response modifiers."*

Despite her determination to oppose traditional medicine, Lydia had to admit that her interest was piqued. With Dee's help, she wrote to Dr. Gordon. He'd written her what was probably a form letter, but it was encouraging. He, too, had used the word "fortunate" in connection to her particular type of cancer.

And a few weeks later, Lydia had found herself in Dr. Gordon's new Georgia office, being interviewed by a nurse.

She hadn't known whether to answer the nurse's questions honestly, that she felt lousy, or pretend that she felt better than she actually did, so they'd be assured she wouldn't drop dead right in the middle of testing their new treatment. She opted for the truth, simply because she didn't have the energy to lie. And so she had told the nurse that the pressure in her chest was persistent and unbearable, that her back pain was agonizing and that she had absolutely no strength left.

The nurse had wanted to know why, if she felt so badly, she wasn't receiving any treatment. And so Lydia had launched into her litany of treatments, including the chemotherapies and her reactions to them, and her experiences with more unconventional approaches. The nurse seemed to be very understanding of her reluctance to undergo further treatment. She was certainly an improvement over Dr. Fremont's grinning idiot assistant.

And at the end of Lydia's tale, despite the horrors she had already endured, the nurse had asked her if she'd be willing to try yet another drug regimen, this one a very new one. From what Lydia had written to Dr. Gordon, the nurse said, she seemed to be highly qualified.

"Highly qualified!" Lydia had blurted. What was this, a contest or a job interview?

But the nurse was quite serious. Lydia had a drug- resistant, disseminated lymphoma that had been developing for a very long time, and despite her complaints of pain and fatigue, Lydia appeared to be in fairly good general health.

She was, in short, a "good candidate" for experimental treatment.

Lydia, after hearing her deadly disease described so positively, couldn't help but laugh. She laughed then cried. In spite of her negative chemotherapy, she found herself signing up for Dr. Gordon's program and making arrangements to enter the hospital for two days of preliminary testing.

It wasn't until she was out in the hallway that she realized that she didn't even know the nice nurse's name. And that she hadn't seen any sign of the mysterious Dr. Gordon.

And so now here she sat, in the hospital bed, waiting for Dr. Gordon. There was a knock at the door. When Robert Gordon opened the door to room 215, he saw a rather tired-looking, middle-aged woman sitting up in bed, thumbing through what appeared to be a textbook.

"Hello, Ms. Green. I'm Dr. Gordon. How are you today?"
"Hi. Okay, for the moment. I think I may need to have my

lungs drained again soon though," she said with some effort.

"We'll see about that. After we've talked for awhile and after my examination and tests are complete, I want to talk to you about your treatment. There are some new drugs I'd like you to try."

"New? What does new mean? New for me, or new to medicine?" Lydia asked. Dr. Gordon hadn't expected quite that question. "Well, each one actually is not new, but their combination, the sequence in which you take them, will be new to you. I've based the regimen on a promising program being conducted at the Federal Cancer Institute. It has worked for a number of their patients. Perhaps it will prove useful for you, too."

"But what makes you think it'll work for me? Nothing else has."

"Like I said, it worked for some patients at the FCI, and most of them had drug-resistant lymphoma like you. It's worth a try." Dr. Gordon continued to go over her history of the disease and completed a detailed examination. When he finished, she continued.

"Tell me more about this FCI place. Is that where the stuff interferon came from a few years ago? And that more recent breakthrough, what was it, interlocking 2 or something like that?" Lydia asked.

"Yes, that's it. And I think you mean the recent trials with Interleukin-2."

"I guess so. Anyway, what is that place?" She knew a great deal about the FCI, having been refused access earlier, but she wanted to hear Dr. Gordon's opinion.

Dr. Gordon pulled over a chair from the other end of the room and sat next to Lydia. She already liked him. She liked the way that he pulled the chair over, suggesting that he was actually going to spend some time just talking with her. And she liked the way that he looked her directly in the eyes; he had nice, comforting eyes. Not like Dr. Fremont who, however competent and caring, had a habit of burying his face in his notes when he couldn't face a not-too-pretty truth or an unanswerable question.

"The FCI is a huge center, where a lot of cancer research is done. They look for cancer causes as well as treatments," Dr. Gordon said. "And they also fund some research programs at various medical centers around the country."

"Who do they do research on? I mean, how does someone like me, who's lived with cancer for 10 years and tried everything from conventional therapies to coffee enemas and apricot pits, get into such a program?" Lydia asked. She was sitting up tall now, although she didn't realize it, looked more animated than she had in months.

"You just apply. Get on a list. Usually your physician makes the referral. And if you have a type of cancer for which they have experimental treatment, they might consider you."

"What are the stipulations?"

"What do you mean?"

"There must be thousands of people with cancer that aren't bad enough to kill them, but are resistant to drugs or radiation or whatever. But I've seen the famous New England Journal of Medicine, heard its studies shouted all over the headlines. Those studies usually have only a handful of people. How do they choose who gets into a program?" Lydia asked.

"There are two other requirements," Dr. Gordon said.

"I thought as much. Money and connections. Or connections and money," Lydia said with a self-satisfied look on her face.

"No," Dr. Gordon responded a bit uneasily. "You must have a prognosis of at least a few months, to give the experimental treatment time to work. And you must be in fairly good physical shape, besides the cancer, of course. Good heart, kidneys, and lungs, that sort of thing. You'd probably do okay on all these counts." He thought of the Interleukin-2 trial that had been announced last month. Those patients had actually been hand-picked for their youth and strength. In fact, to look at them, only an oncologist would be able to tell that they had disseminated cancer. He remembered their response on a recent referral: "We're really looking for the 'perfect patient' for this particular trial. We don't want the treatment to fail." Gordon's patient had been a little too old and a little too sick.

"Still, it just doesn't add up," Lydia continued. What does it cost to get into such a program?"

"Nothing, if you're accepted," Dr. Gordon glanced at his watch, something he did whether he had to be somewhere in particular or not. This patient was really putting him through the ringer. He still had rounds to make, a consult with another patient, a teleconference with a pharmaceutical house, a seminar at 2:00, and a much-dreaded dental appointment at 4:00. He had a great dislike for dentists.

"I still don't see how it can be done," Lydia persisted. Let's say 1,000 qualified patients apply for 20 spots. First come first serve seems a little severe for people with a terminal illness. Do they pick names out of a hat? Take the youngest first?" Lydia pushed on.

"Why don't you write to the FCI and ask them?" responded Dr. Gordon, growing a bit impatient.

"I'll bet if someone had enough money or the right political connections, say a Senator or Congressman, getting into one of those fancy government programs would be a snap," Lydia concluded. "That must happen at least some of the time, doesn't it doctor?"

Dr. Gordon squirmed. He cleared his throat. These questions on political connections were to be avoided. He knew such connections did help at the FCI, but what good would it do to talk to her about it? She was already guessing far too much!

"Ms. Green, we're getting off the topic. I have what I think is a new combination of chemotherapeutic agents that might be effective against your cancer. I know that you've been in a lot of pain, explored a number of different avenues, but, as you've said, you've battled this thing for a long time, so the rest of you must be in pretty good shape. Do you want to give it a try?"

But the questions continued. Lydia was not about to sign herself up for another round of vomiting and hair loss unless she knew precisely what she was getting into. "Will there be vomiting again? And what about my hair?" she asked, diverted finally from her probing questions as she felt her short blond curls.

"I doubt the hair loss will be severe. It is a possibility though," the doctor answered.

"Well, I don't know if I can put myself through all that again. It's worse than the back and lung pain," Lydia said softly.

"Yes, but Lydia -- can I call you that? -- the cancer is spreading. The x-rays we took yesterday showed that. We have to fight it, while we still can. This may be the way."

"So it's more drugs. But there just has to be another way."

They were both silent for a few minutes. Then Lydia continued. "Doctor, I've been thinking. There must be a key to this whole thing in the simple fact that one of four of us gets cancer -- but the other three don't. Why don't they?" She paused. "Do they fight it off somehow" Why can't those FCI hotshots look at healthy people and see what they have that I don't?"

Dr. Gordon was used to cancer patients grabbing at straws, suggesting wild things. But Lydia's perception was indeed remarkable. "Actually, you're suggesting something that scientists have thought about for some time," he answered hesitantly.

"Just thinking about?" Lydia probed again.

"It all has to do with the body's immune system, which we think normally protects a person from infections and perhaps also cancer. And some of the most striking evidence comes not from healthy people, but from some of the most sick people -- AIDS victims, whose immune system breaks down, and organ transplant recipients who are given drugs to suppress their immune system's rejection of the transplanted tissue," Dr. Gordon said.

Lydia was fascinated. "So when the immune system's caught off guard, a cancer can sneak through," Lydia said as she shifted on the bed. "Excuse me. I can't stay in one position for too long because of the pain."

"I know. And you are right about the immune system."

"So, why isn't it being looked at? Or is it? Why are we deluged with these toxic drugs that make hair fall out and rip our guts apart when our own bodies might be coaxed into healing themselves? Why isn't it being done?"

The doctor looked at his watch again, then looked at Lydia's IV drip. "It is. Interferon and Interleukin-2 -- what we call "biologicals" -- are both natural chemicals from the immune system. But the work takes a long time, and as you pointed out, the studies are small, and there are long lists of patients."

"Well, it's good to know that another way is being tried. I only hope that something comes of it in time for me," Lydia said.

"I do too."

An uncomfortable silence filled the room. Dr. Gordon was surprised by the conversation, by the fact that Lydia Green, whether she knew it or not, was second-guessing him, almost reading his mind. If she continued to educate herself about the immune system and cancer -- as her intelligent questions and that text at the bedside indicated she would -- she'd soon piece together the overriding problem in manipulating the immune system to treat cancer. It was a problem of economics, not of biology. The undeniable fact was that each person's immune response and each cancer is unique. That was one reason why a single chemotherapeutic agent or fixed combination against say, breast cancer, failed to help all breast cancer patients. The key to conquering cancer lay in treating each patient like the biological individual that he or she is.

Yes, Lydia might indeed piece this all together, but he hoped that for her peace of mind she wouldn't go from the theoretical, which she could probably understand and handle, to the dollars and cents reality of the situation. That a tailored treatment for each individual might very well be an answer to cancer, but it's not at all an economically feasible venture for a pharmaceutical company that must churn out huge quantities of a substance to turn a profit. The drug industry bitched enough about orphan drugs, those produced for small markets. How could they handle individualized treatments? Unfortunately, access to these treatments would eventually boil down to money.

"So, doctor. Let me think it over. This new chemotherapy, that is."

"Of course. Lydia, I've enjoyed talking to you. I'll stop by tomorrow morning and you can tell me your decision."

"Okay. Thank you. You've given me a lot to think about."

For a few seconds more than was probably necessary, doctor and patient looked into each other's eyes. And each was excited about what might be learned from the other.

Dr. Gordon left the room and Lydia reached for a magazine lying at the foot of the bed. She coughed suddenly, then winced in pain and rubbed the small of her back. She scanned the pages absent-mindedly and was soon asleep, with one hand on her stomach and the other clutching her hair.

CHAPTER 2

RISE TO THE TOP

January 1979

Stephen sank into his plush, overstuffed chair and looked around his comfortable office. By government standards, it was quite large and, although plainly furnished, reflected the accomplishments of his career. The far wall was covered with his many diplomas, awards, plaques and other accolades. To the right of his desk, the bookshelf was crammed full of scientific tomes, a few lay books, and two neat piles of his favorite medical journals, Journal of Clinical Oncology and New England Journal of Medicine. He had two copies of each of the more than twenty books to which he had contributed. To the left of the desk, a small couch, a coffee table, and a trio of standard issue government chairs were arranged for informal conferences. A not-too-attractive wall tapestry was tacked behind the couch, obviously a masterpiece done by a well-meaning but none-too-talented friend or family member.

Stephen turned to look out the large window behind his desk. Although it was only 6:00 P.M., the typical mid-January darkness had fallen over the Federal Institutes of Health (FIH) campus. The lollipop-shaped lights that dotted the campus cast an eery glow on the lines of physicians, researchers, technicians, nurses and ancillary personnel scurrying to begin the nightly trek to their neat little houses in the suburbs. Stephen thought they looked a little like lemmings, and wondered why so many people could commute for an hour or more twice a day, five days a week, seemingly forever.

His way made much more sense. But of course, being Stephen Musso, it could be no other way. He had found an inexpensive but attractive apartment conveniently close to the Federal Cancer Institute (FCI) to make "work" literally a home-away-from-home, not to mention a nice place to entertain promising new female associates. Linda and the kids lived out in the Maryland countryside, like so many of those commuters, in a rambling colonial on an acre of land. But despite the beauty of the suburbs, Stephen chose to stay close to work, close to the web of power and control that he had woven so meticulously.

Stephen stretched out his legs, put them on the desk corner and leaned back in his chair. No standard issue government chair, this one he had specially ordered to soothe his body while he exercised his ever active mind. On this January evening, he was reflecting over the day's activities. Typically, he had been in one meeting after another, flitting from a group of FCI scientists to some university researchers gathered from around the country, then back again to the in-house people.

It wasn't easy to deal effectively with the two groups. The FCI scientists are government employees who recognize the value of resources sent their way. They will do most anything if they think it will enhance their laboratory or their controllable world. The university contingent wants money and power from the FCI, and political influence is used to get them. Each group pushes their pet project -- the FCI scientists constantly striving for larger labs, more technicians, the latest in microscopes, scanners and cell culture innovations, more beds for clinical studies, and in general, a larger slice of the government research pie; the university scientists seek the same, but often garnered recognition from the all-powerful FCI through political means and lobbying, although technically the way to obtain research support funds was to write a grant proposal, and pass peer review.

How naive, Stephen thought, for those who still think that a grant is awarded on scientific merit alone. He thought back to the committee meeting where Dr. Murman, the cell biologist from Wyoming, presented his grant proposal. Although the experimental protocol was straightforward and rather innovative, both Murman and Stephen knew that the fate of the grant had been sealed a week earlier, when a quiet visit had made clear to Stephen that unless this grant was given favorable consideration, the vote of the Senator from Wyoming on the new FCI appropriations bill was in jeopardy.

Stephen took a moment and reflected on his career, a frequent habit that gave him comfort and renewed his motivation to move ahead. Who would have expected this chubby Italian boy to grow up to head the largest division in the FCI? From his position as Director, Division of Cancer Therapy, he had control over $170 million of taxpayer money. He remembered how tough it was to influence friends and associates as a young researcher, and thought how easy it was now to wield influence through this awesome budget. With just a change of expression, a verbal slight, a theatrical gesture in front of a large audience, or a direct written rebuff, Stephen could personally sound the death knell for any researcher's project that fed off of that budget. It was public money but personal power. It had been a long rise to the top, but Stephen knew there was one more step.

Stephen's ultimate goal was no less than the directorship of the FCI. As he looked out over the largest biomedical research complex in the world, Stephen thought his journey was almost over -- one more goal, one more appointment, and one more step to achieve ultimate power.

The current director, Jacob Poldosky, was a wishy-washy wisp of a man who Stephen didn't much like. The man couldn't make decisions, and didn't know Stephen's kind of loyalty to friends and associates when previous favors had been done. He would change positions on the issues when new information became available, and he was much less likely to reward those who helped him and punish those who didn't than Stephen would have liked. Not at all the sort of man to really take charge of this Institute, Stephen thought out loud, but it won't be long, not with this recent information...

There was a soft tap on the door and it opened slightly as Melody, Stephen's administrative assistant, peeked in.

"I'm leaving for the night. Will you need me this weekend?"

Stephen thought a little too literally about her question, but responded, "No Melody, you go on home and have a good weekend. The Federal Cancer Advisory Board meets next week and I have a lot of work to do to prepare for that meeting. So rest up. You and I may have some late nights next week."

A faint smile crossed Melody's lips as she unconsciously twisted a strand of her long dark hair. Was Stephen just imagining a look of anticipation on her face when he mentioned the late nights? But she responded as noncommittally as he had. "Good night and have a nice weekend."

Melody was a lissome young woman in her late twenties, ten years younger than Stephen. They worked well together, and she had the uncanny ability to make him relax, often even laugh, which was much needed in his position. There was clearly an attraction between them, but so far neither had pushed the relationship to anything more than a friendly working association. It was hard for Stephen to tell if a woman really was interested in him, or was just awed by his importance in the organization. Sort of like a rock star, he thought.

After Melody left, Stephen continued to gaze out the window, his thoughts taking him back to childhood. His mother, an immense woman, bore the verbal ravages of his father's frequent drunken rages. To young Stephen, his mother was a saint, always there when he needed her. She cooked, cleaned, took in odd jobs from neighbors and friends, and always had a big hug when the day was rough on a little boy.

The boy felt the underlying conflict between his parents. Although he often comforted his mother when she was crying, they never openly discussed the ever-present strain. His father, as far as he knew, was not physically abusive, he was clearly an intolerant bully to both his wife and child, constantly demonstrating his need to be "the boss".

Vito Musso was a big, burly truck driver, a teamster, and most importantly, a man. He needed to be masculine, being someone whom "nobody could push around", as he often muttered to himself. So it went, day after day, driving 10 or more hours in New York City, then hitting his familiar bar for beer, some casual roughhousing, and an occasional serious altercation.

And the days grew into the years of Stephen's childhood. He hoped his father wouldn't come home. Vito began to work less and drink more. The only constant in his life seemed to be his continually fighting, in bars and at home. So it wasn't too much of a shock when he was found one night beside his truck in Brooklyn. Nothing clean like a bullet or a knife, but beaten and clubbed and stomped. Dental plates were used to identify the body. What Stephen remembered most clearly about the funeral was the undertaker whispering to a cousin what a hard time it was to make his father's body appear presentable. To this day all Stephen needed to do was to think of a funeral, and his father's bloated, purple face would flash before him, the large rough features no longer sharply chiseled.

The contrast between Vito and Patrick was striking. Patrick O'Leary was head of the New York Teamsters union. Although he was an Irishman, Patrick had thin features with prominent cheek bones, a shock of well arranged red hair, and a few freckles across his forehead. Actually, Stephen looked more like Patrick than Vito, with his tawny hair and aquamarine eyes -- only his nose gave away his Italian ancestry.

Educated and outwardly genteel, underneath it all, Patrick O'Leary was clever and uncompromising. After all, as he often told the young Stephen, you don't run a teamsters union in New York unless you know how to do business. And business in the teamsters included money, influence, power and, when necessary, violence. Patrick knew how to use them all.

Stephen remembered the teamsters hall with those loud and boisterous men, knocked about from a day at work and drunk from the evening at the bar. As a teenager he was a yard helper for Action Trucking Lines in Brooklyn. His experience on the job and the counseling by his "foster father" Patrick were to be of continuing value in forming Stephen's outlook on life, although his eventual career would lead him far from the Teamsters and the grimy streets of Brooklyn. The name of the game was power, Patrick told his eager protegee over and over. And power worked best if it was doled out carefully in the form of rewards and punishments. What worked in the teamsters also worked for science, as Stephen would learn.

But sometimes, someone just had to be gotten rid of, even if he didn't deserve punishment. This was the situation now between Stephen and Jacob Poldosky. Quite simply, Stephen could not ascend to the directorship until Jacob moved on. And he now had the power to hasten that move, using some dirt he'd secured last week from an underling in a chemical company. Stephen had helped to secure a government contract for the man and now he owed him something. Now, if he could just get a little more information...

The door suddenly opened with a knock, and Roger Salla strode in. Roger never just entered a room, he bolted into it.

"Hi Stephen. I've got two interesting pieces of news. First, I've discovered a new virus. It's linked to non- Hodgkin's lymphoma."

"What do you mean 'linked'?"

"I mean we have been able to see the virus in the lymphoma cells from one of the patients and we believe it is now growing in tissue culture. You should see the electron micrographs, they are remarkable."

"That's great news, but remember the last time," Stephen cautioned.

"Dammit Stephen, every time I come in here with something new, you bring up 'the last time'!"

"Roger, I'm going to keep bringing it up until you do something to repay me for it. You suffered, I suffered, our whole group suffered from your mistake. I don't ever want to have to explain that kind of mistake again. That faux pas damn near cost me my job and you know it almost cost you yours now, what's the evidence that this virus is real, and not just another contaminant like that last one?"

"Stephen," Roger said excitedly, "this virus was isolated directly from a fresh biopsy specimen, and the cultures were handled only by my chief technician, whom I trust implicitly. Last time I wondered if someone dumped some baboon virus into the tissue culture flask just to throw me off. This time I made damn sure nobody handled those flasks but people I trust. This virus is really it. It's right out of those cells and I believe we've got a potential Nobel Prize."

"Well, I'm just warning you, keep it under wraps until you are absolutely certain. We can't afford another major screwup from your lab. After all, you get more research money now than anybody else. If you expect to keep that kind of support -- no more mistakes. Now, what's your second piece of news?"

Roger smiled crookedly. "I've just had a call from Bill Torbin over at the American Chemical Company. Remember him?"

"Of course I remember him," Stephen said impatiently. "I've been waiting for the past three weeks for the additional information you promised. Come on, what's the story?"

Roger sat down, pulled out a filtered cigarette, and drew in a long, deep breath.

"Roger, will you quite smoking those goddamned cigarettes!"

"Stephen, get off my back. You know viruses are the major cause of cancer," laughed Roger. "Anyway, Bill tells me he has been able to pull out the file on Jacob. It seems that there was a "consulting fee" given to our noble leader during his first year as FCI Director. Supposedly, that fee was for consulting activities with American before becoming director here. In fact, the file shows very little actual consultation, and what's more, the fee was not delivered until nine months after Jacob's appointment as director. Bill thinks a General Accounting Office (GAO) investigator reviewing this file would come to the conclusion that the money was given for influence rather than services."

Stephen leaned forward in his chair, his usually fair face darkening and contorting into the expression that those who knew him well immediately recognized -- the expression of greed and of the need for more power. "How do we get hold of this file, Roger? What does this guy want?"

Roger leaned back. "Well, Stephen, we all want something now, don't we? You want the file, I want a bigger lab and now that Bill has the FCI contract approved, he wants a recommendation for promotion within his company."

"So what does that all add up to?" snapped Stephen.

Roger smiled broadly. "I would like to have the Laboratory of Experimental Virology merged with my own. I want to be chief of a newly reorganized group that controls all those resources. That's all."

"Damn it Roger, we just reorganized your laboratory six months ago! People are going to start griping if I reorganize your lab again and give you still more people." He paused for a moment to think. "I'll tell you what. Be patient and wait for six to eight more months, I believe I can get the head of that laboratory to resign. If so, it will be easier to make the move you're suggesting."

A brief sense of sheer pleasure, almost sexual, passed through Roger. Finally, to be rid of George Trumpey, who heads that laboratory. The end of a long battle. But Roger retorted, "Six to eight months? But George may discover another virus in cancer cells before I do! I need more manpower NOW!"

That dark, intense look again flickered across Stephen's face, but this time, it meant anger. "Roger, I'm telling you one more time. You can have the lab in six to eight months, but if you keep squeezing me on things like this, you're going to have no lab at all one day. Remember, you're part of a family, and you can't ask for more than I can deliver without harming the whole family."

Roger leaned back in the chair, crossed his legs, and slapped his hand on his knee. "Okay, okay. That'll have to do. But what about Bill's needs? Can you get a letter to the VP responsible for the decision to his promotion?"

"Well, his contract is slated for funding. The recommendation letter is no problem. You can tell Bill he is as good as in at American. Now, how do we get to the file?"

Roger got up and jerked open the door. "Bill, can you come on in?" The door opened wider, and a short, rather unkempt man of about 30 entered the room.

"Hello Dr. Musso, I'm Bill Torbin."

Stephen stood up from behind his massive desk piled high with work for the weekend. "Hello Bill, it's nice to meet you. I'm glad to have the opportunity to discuss projects of mutual interest. Roger tells me that you are involved with some very interesting research."

"Yes, we're working to reduce the carcinogenicity of certain chemicals important in the food processing industry. I think we've got some good leads that may prove useful. But it's going to take some action in Congress if we are going to get some of the regulations changed on these chemicals."

"Well, Bill, research is the first step. If you can show good evidence that your point of view is scientifically sound, I think the political action will naturally flow. These kinds of research projects are very high priority with us, you know."

"It's certainly good to hear that, sir."

Stephen sat down and looked sideways at the two men standing before his desk. "Well, have a seat. It's late but maybe we can discuss some of our other business."

Bill sat down and placed a folder on Stephen's desk. As Stephen reached for it, Bill said, "I think you will find the information satisfactory." He paused while Stephen scanned the documents, then added, "Obviously, if anybody finds out that I copied that information, I'm finished."

"Bill, you don't need to worry about disclosure. No one will every know how I received these papers."

Stephen was no stranger to the fine art of blackmail. As he flipped through the folder, he remembered vividly a similar episode that had taken place just two years earlier.

Roger Steel had been in this chair, and Stephen had been head of a smaller clinical group in the FCI. Dr. Steel was a vibrant man, well respected within the research community and innovative in developing new chemotherapies for cancer treatment. His position was rock solid, and there were no clouds on his career horizon.

But he was in Stephen's way.

Two years ago, Stephen had sat in the very chair now occupied by Roger Salla and simply said, "Bob, I have worked for you for more than five years, and I'm sure you're aware that we've had many differences. It's time for me to move on."

"What precisely do you mean?" asked Bob, surprised at the possibility that Stephen, widely-known for his ambition, would be leaving FCI. Many researchers would mortgage their mothers to have his job.

"Let me put it more specifically. It's time for me to replace you!"

Stephen had planned those words for so long that to this day, he could recall the conversation verbatim. The broad smile that had crossed Bob's face at this announcement was not surprising. Laughing, Bob told Stephen what he could do with his proposal. He certainly had no intention of leaving his prestigious post for some aggressive, over confident jerk. But Stephen was prepared. He gave his superior a folder that had taken him months to prepare. Steel still wasn't taking him seriously, but he would in about thirty seconds.

Bob Steel was happily married, with three children and another on the way, the epitome of the American family man. But that image was shattered by the contents of Stephen's mysterious folder -- numerous photos of Bob being more that a little friendly with his secretary, a hot-looking redhead (and a natural one at that) who wasn't quite bright enough to know when to lock a door. Bob's face turned about as red as his lover's hair, his jaw clinched, his fists tightened. He looked straight at Stephen and bellowed, "You arrogant son of a bitch! This is the lowest form of blackmail! I knew you were ruthless, but I never suspected that you would try this!"

It took a while for Bob Steel to realize that Stephen was deadly serious. What sickened him was not so much what Stephen had done, but how he had done it, so cunningly, and so without feeling. Stephen had learned from Bob, had tapped his brain, and when he could learn no more, the next move was obvious -- move up.

From across his desk, Bob Steel had appeared to have aged about ten years, his hair frazzled, his skin drooping, his eyes sad. He had honestly thought that scientific research was somehow immune to this sort of thing. After twenty years of work for the government, he was being forced out by a monster who had no qualms about using a single episode of drunkenness and bad judgement to ruin an honestly built career.

Bob had asked Stephen for some time to think, just a week, but the bastard wouldn't even give him that. He demanded a public resignation the next day, or the folks at the FCI would have some very interesting snapshots to chat about.

"Well," Stephen muttered as he came back to the present and the American Chemical file on Jacob. "This information is certainly interesting. Gentlemen, I believe we have concluded our business. Bill, we will be in touch. Keep up the good work. Roger, can you wait just a moment?"

"Thank you Dr. Musso, I look forward to hearing from you soon."

As Bill Torbin left, Stephen motioned for Roger to check the door. He looked to see that Bill had gone from the outer office and down the hall, returned to the office, and closed the door behind him. "Roger, this information should do the job. I'll move on it quickly. Once Jacob resigns, we'll have control of the whole Institute."

"When do you think we should make a move?" Roger asked. "Oh, it can't be done immediately. I'll have to spend some time behind the scenes. But you can help in the meantime. When old Jacob leaves, I want there to be a natural groundswell of interest in appointment me as director. Now that's going to take some work. I'll be talking to you about some assignments, but for now, I'll just keep this file available for the right moment."

Roger stifled a yawn and Stephen said, "Yes, it's been a long day. I'm going to head for the apartment to do a little reading." Stephen began to arrange some papers to take with him and Roger turned to leave. Then Stephen looked up, "Oh, I almost forgot. Please send me the data on your new virus. Don't make any public disclosure until we've had a chance to talk about it. This time I want to be absolutely certain that you have the virus."

Somehow Roger expected what was coming next.

"Of course you and I will both announce the discovery... if there is one. Given the success of my ABC regimen in lymphoma, you know I have a major interest in related developments. I want to make sure this virus is real and that it's publicized in the right way."

Roger nodded, knowing full well what that meant. Stephen would be a part of the publicity, a co-author on the work, an upfront person taking credit for having provided the resources to Roger. He'd be recognized as the co-discoverer of the virus, although he actually hadn't stepped one foot into the lab where the work had been done. Roger was irritated but he had been through this before with Stephen and others at the FCI. It was the way science was done here -- share the glory to keep the bucks flowing in. The important thing was that he, Roger Salla and not Stephen Musso, would be the first author, and he would be the one to be awarded the Nobel Prize. After all, they give the prize to the scientist, not to an administrator or clinician like Stephen, no matter how powerful he was. So let

Stephen participate, let him co-discover and publicize. The Prize would still come to him!

"Okay Stephen, whatever you say." Roger, ever the gentlemen, shook hands and bounded out of the room much as he had entered it. He walked down the hall thinking Stephen was a real son of a bitch. But was he really any worse that others at the FCI? Even himself? We come from different backgrounds, Roger thought, but Stephen's insatiable thirst for power and recognition were not so different from his own dreams of scientific achievement. The difference was that Stephen didn't care who he had to step on to accomplish his goals. Roger punched the elevator button a little too hard, and, when the doors opened, left the floor where Stephen reigned supreme.

May 5, 1979

The room was brightly lit, uncomfortably so. Standard issue table. Dr. Paulo Brisella, his overweight body stuffed into the cheap government orange plastic chair, sweated profusely from anxiety. He knew a confrontation was coming. He could hear his heart pounding against his chest.

Stephen Musso and one of his henchmen, Sam Fish, quickly entered the room. They were talking rapidly to finish up business from a previous meeting. Both walked over to Paulo and shook hands, murmuring greetings. The three of them sat around the conference table, while coffee was served by a rather unattractive GS7 clerical worker.

In an attempt to overcome his nervousness, Paulo concentrated on the GS7, who was rattling the dishes. She, too, must be nervous, he thought. What happens to ugly GS7s? Do they metamorphose into attractive GS13s? Musso's Melody sure was a looker. Paulo briefly fantasized Melody in the nude. Achieving a GS13 level was a sort of right of passage, for these were the administrative assistants to the brass of the Institute.

Just what was the difference between a clerical worker, a secretary and an administrative assistant anyway? Who cares, they're all the same. Paulo continued to stare at the young woman, avoiding the piercing glare of Stephen.

"Paulo, how is your work going?" asked Stephen.

"Very well. I think we have made some recent observations that will prove very interesting," Paulo said.

"What do you mean?" Stephen asked.

"Well, as you know, we have been working on some improvements for your ABC regimen and we have added some drugs which I think may improve its efficacy in treating lymphoma."

"So I understand," sneered Stephen. "And you've done this without discussing the research with me. Am I right?"

"But Stephen," Paulo whined, "You're a co-investigator on all of our work. We were simply trying to make some preliminary headway so we could show you the results. Then we planned to ask you to help us publish the material."

"Paulo, this is the third time we've had this kind of meeting. The first time involved the publication of some results with a regimen which you thought might supplement or even replace ABC. You know what an unpopular decision that was. Even though you subsequently clarified your position and demonstrated your regimen was inferior, it has always been a sore point for me. You then attempted this recent direct request to Jacob asking for a separate Task Force outside of my division. Jacob didn't grant your request, it was a dumb move. This latest work on additions to my ABC regimen is the final straw." Stephen paused to down his coffee before it got cold.

Paulo fidgeted, making annoying squeaking sounds as he pulled his sweaty arms away from the sides of his chair. "What does that mean?" Paulo asked in a voice that did not quite sound like his usual baritone.

"I'm asking for your resignation." He paused for effect. "If you choose not to give it, I will see that you never have another professional opportunity in the academic community."

Stephen leaned back to let his statement sink in. He could see the disgusting rivulets of sweat all over whatever was exposed of Paulo's corpulent form, and the dark stains it caused on his shirt. Why on earth didn't the pig exercise regularly? The entire scene -- the bright lights, the round table and the orange chairs, brought to mind a similar meeting more than a year ago, when he had met with Drs. Adrian Free and Thomas Frederick.

Known affectionately to the younger investigators as the "F&F twins", Adrian and Tom were co-workers in the development of the ABC regimen. In fact, Adrian had published the first abstract which was appropriate, since the ABC regimen was proposed by Adrian, approved by Tom and himself, and worked on initially by a handful of others, including Paulo Brisella.

That meeting had been interesting. Adrian, Tom, and Stephen had been more or less equals until then, all senior investigators at the FCI. Each had an illustrious career with good academic training at major universities: Adrian at Harvard, Tom at Hopkins, and Stephen at Cornell. The three researchers had been frustrated by the difficulty in maintaining remission induced by a single chemotherapeutic agent. It was clear that the next step was to try drug combinations. What was needed was the RIGHT combination.

With the ABC regimen, Adrian Free's baby, a combination chemotherapy for long-term remission of lymphoma was finally at hand. But the initial abstract authored by Adrian was overlooked because it was presented at the annual meeting of a newly-organized medical oncology society. There was no news or publicity about the original observation. However, all three physicians knew the potential impact of their findings.

Although Adrian had the exceptional scientific insight that led to the development of the ABC regimen, it was Stephen who had the political savvy to hype the work, and twist it to his own benefit.

Before word had gotten around the cancer community about the ABC work, Stephen became head of cancer therapy at FCI. Now he needed something to boost his importance, to demonstrate to the public that his recent rise had been well deserved, and that he would, in time, go even farther up the FCI ladder. And a key to his success would be the ABC regimen.

He had called Adrian and Tom into his new plush office on the afternoon of the morning announcement of his new appointment. Adrian and Tom had also been up for the position, but had accepted Stephen's victory well. They were more than a little curious about the meeting.

After coffee and some inane chitchat about the weather, Stephen handed each of his co-workers a report, himself the first author. It was a new protocol for the treatment of lymphoma. Adrian and Tom glanced through the pages, and immediately realized what Stephen had done, although they could scarcely believe it. The "new" protocol was a precise replica of the original ABC regimen, except that one drug had been changed. The report claimed to be "the new protocol with which all patients with lymphoma would be treated." And as if to justify his action, Stephen had predicted that the new drug regimen would be much more effective than any previous treatment.

But Adrian and Tom couldn't be snowed, as Stephen hoped the rest of the world would be. At first they protested mightily. Stephen, of course, won. He was the director and in a government research institution, the director always wins. The "new" ABC regimen, properly trumpeted to the FCI and the press by Stephen, was a resounding success, a "miracle cure", the Washington Post had said. A 60 percent response rate with most of the patients cured was certainly an advancement. The treatment that made it into public awareness was hailed as a "remarkable discovery and a monumental achievement" by Dr. Stephen Musso. The F&F twins had managed to get their names on the paper, but the name in lights was Stephen's, and Stephen's alone.

Stephen's mind returned to the sweaty Paulo. "Well, Paulo, help me understand why you continue to try to improve on my work without my advice or consent?"

"Stephen," said Paulo, "you know we are friends and have worked together for a long time. I'm not trying to circumvent you or your program, I'm just trying to expand your work. You've been a co-author on everything I've done and you always will be. It is not my intent to hurt you. I want to continue to help you and the Institute."

Stephen smiled, and his eyes narrowed as he glanced obliquely at Fish. "I wish I could believe you, Paulo, I really wish I could. Unfortunately, I'm afraid you have become a dangerous man. There is much I won't divulge, but it is clear that you don't have my best interests at heart. The time has come to make a decision."

Paulo knew he was the only member of the original ABC team still at the FCI. He was the junior author on the original paper and participated in many of the discussions between Adrian, Tom and Stephen. He was well aware that he knew too much. Stephen was about to extinguish the last remaining person with whom he should rightfully share credit for ABC.

"Stephen, what do you want? What can I do to make things right?" Paulo pleaded. "You know the Institute has been my home for ten years, you know I have no interest in going to the university and you know I love this area. What can I do?" he implored.

And as always, Stephen had a "solution." "Paulo, don't worry. You will soon be offered a position at Maryland State University. So you can stay close to what you love. Your family won't need to move, and you can continue your research," said Stephen a little too smugly. "Charles Hunter, the recently deceased oilman, put a large sum in trust to support cancer research at MSU. Perhaps you will find the gift of assistance will offset the sorrow of your departure from the FCI."

"But Stephen, I don't like MSU. I don't really like the people there, and I want to remain at the FCI." whined Paulo, close to tears.

"Paulo, don't make things difficult for me. There are other avenues available, but none as desirable. If you force me into action, many problems will follow, some over which I have no control. My advice is to take this opportunity. Everyone will view it as a promotion."

Paulo looked as if he would soon drown in sweat. He knew he was trapped, and took on that hounddog look of defeat that Stephen savored so. Now all he wanted to do was to get out of there, to get some air. "Stephen, may I have some time to think about our conversation?"

"Sure Paulo, take all the time you need. Talk to your friends and associates about this opportunity, and get some feedback. Let me hear from you within a month."

Paulo rose to leave the room, aware that his chair was soaked. Stephen ignored Paulo. He was trying to figure out how this departure would allow him to do the internal shifting necessary to expand his lymphoma work. Stephen was immensely challenged by manipulating people -- almost as much as he once was by research.

CHAPTER 3

TOP DOG

August 12, 1979

It was hot in Washington but this August was especially unbearable. Controversy was in the air -- politicians accused of using influence for personal gain, Defense Department contracts under investigation for alleged payoffs, and perhaps worst of all, at least for the FCI, headlines in the Washington Post shouting the high risk of cancer from chemicals in our food chain and environment. It seemed as though every day a new cancer-causing chemical popped up in coffee, hotdogs, hamburgers, hair spray, even in the water supply. The flood of letters to the FCI and calls to the cancer hotline were becoming overwhelming.

The heat was on at the FCI and that heat fell directly onto the shoulders of Jacob Poldosky. Jacob was a world-reknowned expert in chemical carcinogenesis. When not in his laboratory -- something unusual for an administrator of his rank -- he could be found in the library pending editorials for medical journals, or in Congressional meeting halls discussing the problems of chemicals in our environment as potential causes of cancer. Poldosky's name often came up in the press when cancer-causing chemicals hit the headlines, and he was well-liked in the media and the scientific community.

The great interest in chemicals as a cause of cancer had peaked in the late 1970s and had contributed to Jacob's appointment in 1975 as FCI director. There was no doubt that Jacob knew a great deal about chemical carcinogenesis. He also knew a great deal about human behavior, and disquieting thoughts about Stephen Musso were bombarding his consciousness of late. There was nothing specific, just Stephen's angular smile, his insincere handshake, his forced conversation. There was something sinister about the man lately. And those Post stories targeting various chemicals and the reporters' insistent questioning of FCI officials added to his disquietude. Something was definitely up.

And the Federal Cancer Advisory Board (FCAB) meeting last week had been strange too. Stephen suddenly spoke at length about chemical carcinogenesis, something that was clearly out of his territory. But one thing Stephen did know was that tomorrow's headlines often originated in today's FCAB meeting.

The FCAB was composed of eminent scientists and well-informed laypeople, who advised the FCI director and the President's Cancer Advisory Panel on the problems of cancer. Since the creation of these bodies by President Nixon's National Cancer Act in 1971, the realities of the FCAB and the President's Panel were ever present. There were those who served in the highest interest of science, and a sincere desire to translate research findings into effective action. There were others who participated for personal, and often political, reasons.

Last week's FCAB meeting was typical. A round table, a group of top scientists and a contingent of well-respected lay individuals, all pressing for attention, and the gallery for observers, populated by interested FCI employees as well as by the press. Some of the observers were there to learn and to provide information to others. Most were there for enjoyment, to watch the circus of Dr. X nailing Dr. Y, with Dr. Z auguring for attention.

Each of the directors had made his report. Stephen's had been unexpected. He seemed to be making the point that certain chemicals were more suspect as cancer-causing agents than had earlier been thought. Stephen, head of cancer therapy, normally had little to say about cancer causation or about chemical carcinogenesis. Nonetheless, he discussed specific chemicals that might be especially dangerous. These statements were made when the Washington Post series was very prominent in everyone's mind. Jacob thought it curious that Stephen's statements coincided with the newspaper series in citing certain chemicals, which were not previously considered to be particularly worrisome.

Jacob also noticed with some alarm that Stephen mentioned specifically the American Chemical Company. Jacob had previously done some consulting for this company, and he wondered now if there might be some connection with Stephen's discussion. But at the meeting, Stephen had simply come to the conclusion that we needed to look carefully at our environment and our industries for evidence of cancer causation, and perhaps be more sensitive to the presence of these chemicals as potential carcinogens. It seemed innocuous on the outside, but Jacob couldn't help but wonder what was churning in Stephen's devious mind.

While Jacob was mulling over the FCAB meeting, Stephen, one floor below, was having similar thoughts. Jacob's office was directly above Stephen's, and more spacious. Whenever Stephen visited, he mentally rearranged the furniture and replaced the trappings with his own.

As he returned to his office, he called Sam Fish.

"Sam, I want you to keep feeding information to the Post on chemical carcinogenesis."

"Okay, sure Stephen. But how far do I go?"

"Sam, I don't know for sure, but I want the series to continue. Keep the reporter interested. More to come later!"

"Sure Stephen. Whatever you say."

Sam's a good man, Stephen thought. He does what he's told with minimal questions, doesn't ruffle feathers, and gets the job done. He knew many FCI scientists liked Sam because of his flexible approach to everything, but others called him a mealy-mouthed ass-kisser. He used Fish to send up trial balloons and get tasks done that he would have been uneasy doing himself. In short, Sam was a quiet and effective hatchet man.

As Sam scurried away to do his boss' bidding, Stephen patted himself on the back for his wise decision to come to the FCI. He had almost gone to Sloan-Kettering, a fine, powerful institution, but in no way comparable to the FCI in terms of respect and political power. He had worked here as a clinical associate, then as a senior investigator, a senior physician leading his own clinical research group, and finally as director of cancer therapy. To most who knew him, he was an innovative and dedicated clinical scientist. Had he not invented ABC? Wasn't that considered the major advance in cancer treatment in the last decade? Never mind that others were involved, Stephen had been the driving force behind the work and he knew that he was recognized as such.

He thought back to his foster father, Patrick O'Leary, who had died recently. Stephen had gone to see him when he was very sick. They sipped coffee together, laughed, and talked about the old times and the Teamsters, of how important it was for people to stick together and help one another. As usual, Patrick had drummed away at loyalty, friends, and family, and how relationships helped to "get things done." For Stephen it was like a refresher course, a trip back in time. Stephen was reminded of the time, long ago, when Patrick had suggested that he drop the final "o" and change the "a" in his given name Stephano, so that he would sound more like a professional and less like the son of an immigrant truck driver. Stephen had followed his mentor's advice, although he hadn't been entirely sure why.

Stephen returned to the present, looking out over the scorching August day. He could see the scientists and technicians scurrying from place to place in casual open- necked attire. He hated hot weather, but his office was cool and comfortable. Maybe he should sleep here, avoiding even the short commute to his apartment. Melody's perfume lingered in the room, and Stephen's hormones were raging. The fragrance, her body, his mind soared. Maybe Melody would stay too...

A sharp rap on the door announced Roger's typically aggressive entrance.

"Stephen, here's the data on the new virus. The experiments are convincing and conclusive. We are ready to publish. I've already written it up, and it goes to Science tomorrow."

Stephen looked Roger squarely in the eyes. "Roger, you will send this to Science when I tell you to, and not before. I want to look the report over and get an outside opinion before Science sees it. You know it will be extensively reviewed anyway. Better to catch the glitches here."

"But, but..." sputtered Roger. His face reddened as he dug in his soiled shirt pocket for a Marlboro.

Stephen interrupted, "Don't worry about credit. I'm going over these results with a fine toothed comb, and make sure that you don't make the same mistake again. The process should take only two or three weeks. You'll just have to cool your heels until then."

Roger looked like a firecracker about to explode. He smoked, he paced, he fumed, he cursed, he was in the chair, out of the chair, while Stephen sat back and watched. More than five minutes passed as Roger stomped back and forth, acting like a child denied a much-wanted toy. Stephen expected him to fall to the floor and throw a temper tantrum. Finally, he began to settle down.

Stephen then said "Roger, you are a great virologist. You have tremendous resources. No one in this country or anywhere in the world has as much support as you do. You have the best people working for you. Surely you can wait three or four weeks so that we can verify that you have made a real discovery. No one is going to scoop you on this."

Finally, the fight was out of Roger. He slumped down in the chair and said, "Okay, I don't like it, but I don't have any choice. But please hurry, because I don't know how close others are to a similar discovery. You know how important this project is to me."

Stephen looked squarely at Roger. "Important to you, your laboratory, and those in it."

Roger's response was immediate, his face contorted like a cocaine addict lusting for a line. "To hell with my laboratory and those in it. This is my work and I'm going to get credit for it. I need it as soon as possible."

December 19, 1979

The time had come.

Stephen was at his desk writing furiously, too busy to join in the holiday festivities around him. He scrawled his name, and sat back and read the note.

"Jacob,
I need to see you as soon as possible, about some recent developments. Could we have dinner together tonight? I'd suggest L'Placio. I know you love Mexican food. How about 8:00? I have already checked with Imogene, and you are free. If we can get together for dinner, I think you will find the meeting of great value."

Stephen jumped up quickly and carried the sealed note out to Melody, who had on a particularly revealing red and beige sweater. "Please take this up to Dr. Poldosky's office as soon as possible. I need to see him tonight."

Melody immediately put aside her work, gave him that ambiguous "can I help?" look and said, "Anything you want, Dr. Musso."

Loyal, dedicated, and beautiful Stephen thought. Probably the best GS13 in the whole government. Before his imagination could run away with him again, he went back into his office and closed the door, an unmistakable "do not disturb" message to the office personnel -- except Melody, he hoped.

Stephen glanced at his desk, piled high with work as usual. Research reports, personnel applications, letters requesting assistance, tons of dictation to do. He was beginning to miss the excitement of science that had originally drawn him to oncology. Lately it seemed to be buried somewhere beneath the continual avalanche of paper. Tonight he just couldn't concentrate on his paperwork. A great confrontation was ahead, the most important of his career, and he was already savoring it.

As Melody made her way upstairs to the FCI director's office, Jacob was working on a book that contained a terrific collection of papers. He was proud to be its co-editor. The many papers and books that he had authored over the years were a great satisfaction to him. They were like his children -- he had created them and continued to love them. The value of education and of intellectual property had been impressed upon him from very early childhood, by his poor immigrant Polish parents. They taught him that intellect was the way to succeed. Although deep down he agreed with this philosophy, he was beginning to see that it wasn't very realistic. The FCI, a center for some of the finest minds in the nation, maybe the world, was at the same time a political hotbed. Over and over again he had seen political manipulation transform what seemed to be a scientifically sound approach to an inferior because it was more politically feasible. Jacob was uneasy with the kinds of pressures that were brought to bear by his friends in Congress, by his colleagues in various universities across the country, and, of course, by his subordinates right here at the FCI.

In addition, the summer's newspaper articles on chemical carcinogens continued to disturb him. Although the series had ended, there were some short footnotes appearing from time to time, and some of those mentioned the American Chemical Company. A few of the items seemed almost deliberate, as if there was some one person planting little tidbits of information with an investigative reporter. These pieces appeared with a certain regularity, a short blip on an inner page of the Post every week or two. They mentioned familiar chemicals and one in particular on which he had done consulting for American prior to his appointment at the FCI. Things were beginning to hit a little too close to home. Jacob had the vague sense that something was snowballing which concerned him, and over which he had no control.

As Jacob was worrying about the mysterious news clip, the door opened and the highest ranked secretary (or was she an administrative assistant) in the FCI entered. Imogene Buchanan had been his secretary since he became director, and she had held the same position with two previous FCI directors. A GS-14 of great capability, she was now in her early 60s and nearing retirement. No beauty, she was a competent manager of the director's affairs. Her many years at the FCI had given her a certain valuable insight into FCI political games. Plus, she knew when to keep her mouth shut. Imogene walked over to Jacob's desk and handed him a folded paper, saying "This just came up from Dr. Musso. Mel said you should read it and respond right away."

"Thanks." Curious. Stephen had never asked him to dinner before, not even to lunch. In fact, they socialized very little, maybe just an occasional drink prior to an official dinner. Jacob had a sense of something about to go very wrong. Why was Stephen being so precise about tonight and why had he gone to the trouble of clearing it with Imogene, who hadn't even recalled Stephen's asking? Had Stephen taken it upon himself to leaf through Jacob's calendar? Jacob picked up the phone and dialed Stephen's extension.

"Stephen, Jacob here. I do have other plans for tonight. Can dinner wait?"

"I'm afraid not. I have some information that I think you will want to see, and I believe that any delay would not be in your best interest." Stephen said, intentionally mysterious.

"May I ask you just what this is all about?"

"I would rather save it for tonight. It's not something we should talk about over the phone."

Jacob sighed. "Okay, I'll see you at "L'Placio at 8:00. Perhaps we can have a brief dinner and finish by 10:00."

"No problem. We can easily complete this matter over dinner."

Jacob hung up and tried to turn his attention to the papers on his desk, but he couldn't concentrate. What on earth did that scoundrel want now?

Stephen was sitting quietly at the bar at L'Placio nursing his second scotch on the rocks. A striking blonde walked in and for a moment he thought it was Connie.

He'd first noticed Constance Kelley three years ago when she was a technician in the tissue culture lab on the seventh floor of building 10. Who wouldn't notice her, with that long golden mane and that chest that entered a room well before the rest of her. By the time she had evolved into a research assistant, he lowered himself to talk to her and found, somewhat to his surprise, that she was both interesting and charming, if not quite a genius. Now that she was assistant to the director of research grants administration, he had come into contact with her more and more often in the past few months. She was making it increasingly difficult for him to concentrate at grant meetings; she was consistently staring at him. Stephen knew that he was attractive but certainly Connie had a stable of horny physicians and administrators chasing after her -- she wouldn't have time for anyone else.

He had been wrong. Connie had had time, and a lot more, for him. He had found out the night before after they had started talking about runaway HeLa cells at a cocktail party and ended up drinking a little too much. They'd helped each other back to his apartment, then to his bedroom. He didn't remember very much, except that she was beautiful and exciting and warm and loving and temporarily made him forget the intensity of his various FCI-related pressures. Maybe the week-long separations from his wife were getting to him. He had behaved like an animal and she was a more than willing partner.

He wondered what Connie had thought of it all. Probably very proud of herself for making it with someone of his stature. Now that he thought about it, she had seemed to be going out of her way lately to stop by his office. Maybe she just honestly liked him, one never knew. At any rate, he knew they probably shouldn't repeat what had happened last night. After all, he was married, and he was mentally nurturing something with Melody. But he also knew that Connie Kelley was completely irresistible, and it would indeed happen again.

Stephen's meandering thoughts were interrupted by a hand on his shoulder. Always courteous, Jacob put out his hand to show the way and said, "Shall we go to dinner?"

Stephen led them to a table in a darkened corner of the small Mexican restaurant. They shared a half-bottle of lightly chilled California Pinot Noir. This was followed by some casual conversation and generous portions of Mexican tortillas filled with a spicy meat sauce and covered with chili beans and sour cream. Both men ravished the food, and washed it down with St. Pauli dark. Each inquired of the other's health, family and activities. And then it was time for business.

With a mug of coffee in his hands, Stephen began, "Jacob, I have come upon some information you will find of great interest." The other man looked nervous. Jacob was glancing about, as if worried that someone might overhear what was about to be said. "Perhaps you have noticed the continuing news reports in the Post on chemical carcinogens?" Stephen continued.

Jacob nodded uncomfortably.

"I'm sure you remember the critical series on the same subject a couple of months ago by Smith and Klinner."

Jacob nodded again, and began to shred his napkin.

"I have recently learned that Joe Smith is interested in this area to a much greater degree than I had previously appreciated. Seems as though he has some information about a certain chemical that may be much more toxic than was formerly thought. My information source tells me that a major story on this chemical will be coming out in the Post in the very near future. It could break within the next two or three weeks."

"How does this concern me, Stephen?" Jacob said guardedly.

"The chemical is three deca-durabrocinic carboxylate or, as it is called by the American Chemical Company, '3-D DDuron'."

Jacob choked on his coffee. He now knew the score. A feeling that had begun weeks ago deep in his gut quickly found its way to his throat, and he began to feel nauseated. The heavy, spicy Mexican food didn't help. The director of the prestigious FCI fought for control. It was still possible that Stephen was bluffing, just pumping him for information to get someone else. He tried for a calm look as he repeated his question, "Yes, but how does that concern me?"

"Jacob, I think you know. You served as a consultant to American shortly before, or perhaps even after, your appointment as FCI director."

"Certainly not after, Stephen, but yes, I did consult briefly with them prior to my appointment here."

"Jacob, I must be very frank with you. I know both the quality and the quantity of consulting you did, and the amount of the consulting fee and the time of payment."

"So?" Jacob said evenly.

"That information may well cause you difficulty, given the size and timing of the fee and the amount of consulting. Over and above that issue, there is the recommendation that you made to American."

Jacob turned red. "Just what do you mean?"

"I mean, and you know, that you were the primary consultant recommending the continued use of 3-D Duron as an insecticide for crops. This is a chemical that Joe Smith of the Washington Post will report to be a highly toxic carcinogen."

"But that information must rest on new findings. And since when do we judge carcinogenicity by a journalist's report?"

"We don't, but the public does. And Joe's articles will rest on findings that you overlooked in your investigations, some of which were published prior to the time of your recommendation. At the very least, your recommendation looks silly in light of Smith's report. The Post articles, combined with the revelation of the size of the consulting fee you received, will put you in an impossible position.

Jacob forced a smile. "Stephen, I doubt this represents a major problem. I certainly don't intend to discuss the issue, and I am sure American Chemical will likewise not be interested in public statements on the matter. Just why are you involving yourself in this anyway?"

"Jacob, let me be very clear and direct. I have worked my way up through the ranks of the FCI from clinical associate to senior investigator to division director. I fully intend to be FCI director. You have done a good job over the past several years, and you can leave with a great deal of respect. I know for a fact that there are many opportunities available to you, one of which is a senior position with your old university. You're 62 and will retire anyway in three years. This represents an excellent opportunity for you to leave gracefully to become a senior scientist at the University of California. Should you choose to follow that course, your future will be assured for the rest of your life."

Stephen paused to let the proposal sink in. Jacob looked impressed, but still a little confused. Stephen saw he would have to spell it out.

"However, should you choose to attempt to stay, I can assure you that there will be a great deal of publicity, at the very least an investigation of your role with American and no doubt a great political problem for you personally and to the Institute. Would you care to see some of the files that Joe Smith has?" Stephen asked as he fingered the confidential reports that Bill

Torbin had ferreted out for him many months earlier. "I think you should think seriously about the California option."

Jacob fought to keep his composure. He wanted to lean across the table and literally crush Stephen's smirking face. A few minutes ago he had merely disliked the man. Now he hated him with a passion he had never experienced before. Never a violent man, Jacob chose words instead.

"I have spent my entire adult life in the service of mankind, in the service of the government, in the service of science. My consulting fee was high, but not outrageous, and my recommendations to American Chemical were made to the best of my knowledge. Perhaps I made an error, but it certainly wasn't a conscious one. Unfortunately, the logic of your presentation is clear, and I am sure that with your help, an investigation would indeed take place. The damage to me, my family and my associates would be irreparable." He paused to maintain his composure. "You are a reprehensible and malicious excuse for a human being, with an insatiable thirst for power. Your time will come, and I hope I am around to see it."

With that, Jacob stood straight and tall, but shaking with rage. He threw the shreds of his napkin into his plate, and stormed out of the restaurant. Stephen waved for the waiter, and enjoyed a second warm mug of coffee.

And so the gears for his final move up the ladder were locked into motion. Next, Stephen thought, would be the task of involving his team completely in the political maneuvering to achieve the directorship. Stephen had of course already done a great deal of homework, and he knew just which buttons to push to bring the unbiased process around to his appointment. He imagined Jacob's resignation would come within the next few weeks. So he had some time to further develop his constituency. Since this was a Presidential appointment, it would be a decision over which he had no direct control.

The rest, of course, is history. On February 2, 1980, Dr. Stephen A. Musso was appointed director of the Federal Cancer Institute. The appointment was hailed as one of the most significant of our time, with article after article recounting his accomplishments, including the discovery of ABC chemotherapy. There were many in Washington who believed that the FCI needed sound management and a major reorganization.

Stephen Musso was just the man to do it.

CHAPTER 4

FALL FROM GRACE

Summer 1980

"Mrs. McNamara, what a lovely family you have? Is that Jason, over there in the corner?"

"Yes. He just loves to look at the big bright pictures in those books. But, of course, he'll probably never be able to read words. He might as well enjoy the pictures."

"Why is that?" asked the reporter, although it was perfectly clear that she knew the answer. The camera zoomed in for a close-up of Joan Archmont's flawless features as she practically shoved the microphone into the mother's face.

"Jason has Down's syndrome." The mother sounded as though she was quite practiced in discussing her son's condition.

"And what does that mean for Jason?"

"It means that he'll never achieve the intellectual milestones that other children will. If he's lucky, maybe someday he can live on his own, perhaps even hold down a menial job of some sort. But for now, all we can do is give him the happiest childhood we can. "Come here, baby," she called as the chubby little boy skipped over to her. "Do you want to say 'hi' to everyone from Television Land?"

"Hi!" yelled Jason, as the camera panned in for a full face shot, a shot held just a little too long, to be sure that the viewers noticed the child's slightly slanted eyes and flattened nose, the visible signs of his Down's syndrome. "Mrs. McNamara, do you have any idea what might have caused Jason's condition?"

"Well, of course I can't prove it - I'm not a doctor - but the answer's obvious to me."

"And that is ..." prompted the reporter.

"Just look at the facts. When we lived in New Hampshire, I had three children - Michael, who's now 17, Christie, who's 14, and Peter, who's 10. Then we move, I get pregnant, and Jason, my fourth child, has this problem. And they have the nerve to tell me it's in his chromosomes! Just look at them over there, playing with their poor brother." Another pan to Jason.

"So you're saying that something about this area - Fairfax, Connecticut - caused your son's defect?"

"Yes," said the mother, a bid subdued.

"What might it have been? Any ideas?"

"You bet. It's that damned plant near the river, dumping God knows what into our water supply. That's what messed up the chromosomes in our family. American Chemical is responsible, that's who."

Fade out, with 30 seconds of footage showing the American plant with smokestacks spewing. Back to the newsroom, and Joan Archmont's mannequin-like face once again. "Let's think about Jason as we hear a word from our sponsor."

Daniel Weil turned the sound down on the remote just as a plastic-looking young woman gaily began to demonstrate the unending virtues of a personal itching preparation. A delightful sight to follow his dessert.

"Come here, Eleanor. I've seen awful news reports before, but this one is unbelievable."

Eleanor Weil put down the silver that she was polishing, and came over to her husband, who looked like he was about to have a stroke. "Dear, I wish you wouldn't get yourself so involved. I do worry about your health, you know."

"How can I not get involved? That's my company they're smearing all over the TV!"

"Well, what is it this time? Toxic leaks again?" Eleanor asked.

"Joan Arch-ass is parading around a poor Down's kid, blaming his condition on our plant. Of course, the mother is such a moron that the kid probably inherited the problem. But on top of that, mom is 45 if she's a day - even announced the ages of her other kids. Teenagers, for Christ's sake. And they blame it on us. But, of course, they 'can't prove anything'," he sneered.

"Dear, please calm down. You won't be able to sleep after this, and you know it will just aggravate your cough. Let's just turn it off - we've heard it all before."

"No. We can't miss the parting cheap shot. Joan's bound to trot out some local leukemia victims next. Or maybe do a miscarriage survey. Let's see now."

Joan Archmont was back. "Poor little Jason. His mother claims to have no proof that American Chemical is responsible for his condition, but I guess we'll never know the whole story. But is it just a coincidence that this county seems to have an unusually high number of cases of childhood leukemia, that the allergy clinics are filled beyond capacity, and that nearly everyone seems to suffer from frequent headaches and even nausea?"

Flash to an on-the-street interview.

"Excuse me. We're conducting an informal survey. Can you tell us how you have been feeling lately?" the reporter said to a fortyish woman in a smart business suit.

"What do you mean?" the woman asked, glancing at her watch.

"Well, some people in the area have noticed increased headaches and fatigue over the past few weeks. And local drugstore merchants report an increase in sales of over-the-counter pain medications. Have you had any health problems?"

"I had the flu two months ago, like everyone else. But yes, now that you mention it, I have been feeling kind of out of sorts lately. Tired. And yes, I've had headaches."

"About when did this start?"

"Just within the past few weeks, I guess. Hey - why are you asking these questions?"

"I'm glad you asked. We're trying to see if there's been a local increase in medical complaints corresponding to the time period over which methylene chloride has been spilling into the river from the chemical plant."

The interviewee looked as if she was about to say something - you could see the word "but" forming on her lips - but smart Joan's microphone was quickly pulled out of sight.

"So there you have it, ladies and gentlemen. Not a scientific survey, certainly, but at least one person has noticed a change in her health since the methylene chloride leak." She paused expertly. "Could there be more like her? Like Jason?"

"This is just too much. That degree of irresponsibility just cannot be tolerated," Daniel muttered as he paced about his spacious living room, shoving his hands in and out of his pockets and repeatedly clearing his throat.

"Dear, you're nearly 80 years old. You mustn't let yourself get so upset. She's not attacking you personally."

"Like hell she isn't. American is me. I built that company. It's as much a part of me as an arm or a leg."

"But what have the real studies revealed? Is there any basis in fact to what that reporter's suggesting?"

"Suggesting? She might as well come right out with an accusation, instead of disguising it. And no, the studies have not shown anything definitive at all. These Down's cases seem to come out of the woodwork whenever there's a spill or leak of some kind. I pity those poor kids, but it's true that where there's a leak, there'll be litigation. Their folks are probably broke from medical expenses, so why not try to drain a corporate giant bad boy?"

"Dear, there's no need to yell," Eleanor said in a deliberately low voice.

Daniel was quiet for a few moments. "I'm sorry," he said, as he hugged his wife. "I get irrational when it comes to this whole mess. But I've done science my whole life. All I ever wanted was to study biochemistry, to see how things work and maybe make life a little better for people, while earning a living," he said in a soft voice that sounded like it was coming from a different person than the one who had been raving just a few minutes before.

"Where did it all go wrong? Where did I go wrong?"

Daniel had loved science for as long as he could remember. And his life had begun in a most unlikely place for the study of things natural.

He was born in 1901 in his parent's sagging bed, which occupied much of one of two tiny rooms located in a tenement on Rivington Street, in the heart of New York City's Lower East Side. In recent years he'd taken to visiting the place of his birth, sneaking downtown from business meetings to walk through the littered streets that really hadn't changed much since the turn of the century. The row upon row of four-story buildings packed along the streets on each side had looked old even when he was a boy, as if they had been built already half-decayed. On his visits, Daniel liked to imagine that he had entered a time machine. The sense of other-worldliness that he remembered from his childhood was still there, that feeling created by people from other lands settling and sharing their customs, their foods, whatever they had brought with them. Or maybe it was just the vivid memory of his childhood that made the dirty streets and old buildings come alive.

The Weils were relatively well-off. Food was always on the table. And Daniel's parents enjoyed the supreme luxury of having their very own tiny bedroom. They had arrived from their shtetl in Rumania at Castle Garden at the southernmost tip of Manhattan island in 1890, just eleven years before Daniel's birth. His mother, an accomplished seamstress, was lucky to have found work immediately, sewing the sleeves onto dresses that she could not afford to buy. She earned $4 a week, but, after paying fees for using the company's needles and electrical power, paid the weekly charge for her locker and tax on the wooden chair she sat on, it was closer to $3. This shrunk even further when she was fined for tardiness.

His father worked in the same factory, carrying bolts of yard goods and matching fabrics and threads. He, too, brought home $4 a week, less usage charges. To supplement his income, Sam peddled straw baskets in the Washington Market every Saturday, adding an extra $4 to the weekly pay if he was lucky. Although Saturday was the Sabbath, money was more important than religion.

And then something happened that was so terrible that Daniel blocked it from his mind - but it would come back to haunt him much later in life.

It was March 25, 1911. His mother was at home because it was the Sabbath, and his father was in Washington Market selling his baskets. Daniel had been reading when he heard a commotion in the street. He raced outside, and followed a crowd to the corner of Green Street and Washington Place. When he saw what was causing the uproar, he stood rooted in place, too horrified to move.

Daniel stood before a 10-story factory building, looking up at the top 3 floors, the Triangle Shirtwaist Company. Flames leapt from the windows of the wooden structure. But what caused the transfixing terror was the people - mostly Jewish and Italian girls in their late teens - who jumped from the windows when the heat behind them became unbearable. Each, in turn, would come crashing down to the pavement, creating a pile of broken bodies. A young man and woman fell to their deaths holding hands. Finally, the firefighters came, but their ladders reached only to the seventh floor.

Daniel saw and heard it all. The fires seared his memory. The bodies broken in the street.

The next day, the Jewish Daily Forward reported 141 identifiable dead, and several bodies burned beyond recognition. The Lower East Side virtually shut down as the people went from one funeral to another. The older people were grimly reminded of the murderous rampages that had driven them from their homelands, but of course the culprit here was an unsafe factory, not stampeding soldiers. All anyone could talk about was the Triangle Shirtwaist disaster. All except Daniel. His 10-year-old mind just could not comprehend what he had seen and heard, and so he simply repressed it.

City College was free to New York City residents, so all Daniel had to come up with was subway fare, which was easy because he kept his part-time job. His parents had put away some money for education, so Daniel could afford books. Daniel truly blossomed in college, studying a variety of subjects. He made friends easily, although he knew that this was helped by his blond good looks and his German-sounding name. Had his new-found friends known where he disappeared to late every afternoon, they might not have been quite as accepting of him in their social circles.

A combination of courses captured Daniel's imagination in his sophomore year - microbiology and chemistry. He eagerly memorized the different classifications of bacteria and protozoa, and he had an intuitive grasp of the interactions between chemicals. What fascinated Daniel, and what his learned professors could not help him to understand, was the gray area between biology and chemistry. Where did the smallest living things overlap with the largest known chemicals? Gradually, over that first semester of his sophomore year, Daniel began to formulate a question that would continue to challenge him, and many others, for years to come. That is, how do chemicals form living matter?

Had Daniel been a child of the 1950s, he would have found his niche in the field of molecular biology that blossomed in the 1970s and 1980s - a field whose entire goal was to dissect the molecules of life, see how they work, and perhaps make them work better. But in the 1920s, the area that Daniel had defined in his head did not exist in university course catalogs.

So he continued to take biology and chemistry, eventually majoring in both. He gravitated more and more to the study of microscopic life, and the study of the more complex organic chemicals. He especially loved the laboratory classes, where he could tear apart bacterial cells to his heart's delight, see what was in them, dump various chemicals on them, observe any interesting results. He imagined himself a creator, chemicals to life forms, by his hands.

It was during the summer between Daniel's junior and senior years that he met Professor Thomas Collins, who taught advanced biochemistry. Daniel wanted to write his term paper for the course on the idea of life's origins from chemicals. But when he went to the library at City College, and then to the one at Columbia, all he found were classifications of microorganisms or proposed structures of molecules.

But Daniel persisted, and wrote his paper without references, because there simply weren't any. It was a gamble, he knew. This was supposed to be a research paper, and he might just be earning himself a D, but he quickly churned out 10 pages of his theories concerning the chemical nature of life.

And he was lucky. He had touched on an area that also fascinated Professor Collins, although he had never mentioned it in class because he correctly thought that most of his students would have enough difficulty in learning the basics, let alone a complex idea that had not yet even been adequately addressed in the scientific literature. He recognized in Daniel Weil a kindred spirit, and offered the boy a dishwasher job in his lab.

Daniel was never one to enjoy dishwashing, but the scrubbing and wiping was tolerable as long as he could listen to the conversations in the lab. There he absorbed more protein chemistry than he ever could have learned in a class. One morning at the start of the spring semester, Dr. Collins mysteriously asked Daniel to see him later that afternoon. Dr. Collins began by asking Daniel his intentions after graduation. Daniel squirmed a bit, and said he really didn't know. Most young men from his background went into the garment industry. But he knew he didn't want to spend the rest of his life inventing the perfect brassiere. Much to his relief, the professor had an idea. Would he consider graduate school - and work in his lab?

In a few minutes, Dr. Collins had outlined Daniel's entire future. First, graduate school, where he'd join the project as an active member and really DO protein chemistry, then perhaps get a faculty position somewhere and start his own research group. And so Daniel applied for admission to the graduate program in Chemistry, and with Dr. Collins backing him, was quickly accepted. They'd even pay him a small stipend for teaching introductory chemistry. No more part-time work in the factory.

For Daniel, graduate school was not much different from his senior year in college. He soon gained a reputation as a brilliant researcher, if a rather sloppy one. The technicians and student assistants were at first annoyed at the mess that he often left in his wake, but his charm and infectious interest in what he was doing, and his desire to explain it to anyone who would listen, won him friends.

He breezed through his qualifying exams at the end of his second year. He could not devote himself entirely to research. Professor Collins - Tom now - had suggested that Daniel branch out from protein chemistry into an area that was even less well studied - hormone secretion involving the hypothalamus and the pituitary.

Daniel was proceeding well, gathering his observations on his pituitary-less mice for his Ph.D. thesis, when he got his first taste of being scientifically scooped. In a 1925 issue of the Journal of the American Medical Association, one P. E. Smith published a detailed account of the effects of pituitary removal on the rat. He noted the same lack of growth, failure to gain weight, loss of libido, lowered disease resistance, loss of appetite and strength and impaired glandular function that Daniel had carefully recorded, but hadn't yet published, in mice. Daniel had been so hell-bent on plunging ahead, learning more and more, that he hadn't stopped to collect his data and publish.

But Daniel's meticulous and accurate work did not go unnoticed by his mentor, who felt a little guilty about not giving his student more guidance in the nuances of scientific publishing. The work also did not go unnoticed by a red-haired stranger who, it turned out, was to profoundly influence Daniel's career.

It was a beautiful fall day in 1926, and Professor Collins and Daniel were talking about their endocrine work at a regional scientific meeting. There were many big names present, but Daniel had not heard of the red-haired gentleman who had asked him several probing questions after his talk. The man, it turned out, was not from a university like most of the others at the meeting, but was a representative of the American Chemical Company, headquartered in Fairfax County, Connecticut. He took Daniel out to lunch, and gradually brought up the possibility of Daniel coming to American after he received his Ph.D.

Daniel at first couldn't imagine why a major chemical company would be interested in someone whose skills consisted of chopping proteins into amino acids and chemically dissecting mouse brains. But after an hour of conversation, his mind was buzzing with all sorts of new research ideas. American was interested in applying information on pituitary functioning to the human reproductive system, with the short-range goal of understanding how human reproductive hormones work, and the long-range goal of controlling fertility, perhaps helping those who couldn't conceive children, or even preventing conception in those who did not want to have any more.

It all sounded quite science-fictionish to Daniel, and in his usual forthright manner, he said so. But the company researcher had gone on about the possibilities in applying basic research in endocrinology to drug development, and Daniel soon found himself caught up in the excitement. The starting salary was most attractive, too. By the end of the lunch, he had made arrangements to visit American's facilities.

He burst into the apartment and immediately launched into a spirited speech on his afternoon meeting. He was so excited that much of it was incomprehensible jargon to his wife. Finally he stopped talking, pleased to see that she looked as breathless and excited as he. He waited for her response.

"I'm sure Daniel, Jr. would just love Connecticut!" Eleanor had answered.

And with that one unforgettable sentence, Daniel's mind was made up. He'd let Dr. Collins try to argue him out of his decision tomorrow, but he knew exactly what he, and his growing family, would do.

Dr. Collins had made a valiant effort to steer his student back on the road to academe. He had already invested several years in leading Daniel to a faculty position of his own, where he would have his own lab and train his own graduate students. The fact that Daniel always had more ideas than he could handle, and that he had a way of looking at problems and envisioning mechanisms that no one else could, would make him an ideal researcher and teacher, Collins thought. And Daniel had seemed interested in following his mentor's academic footsteps too, at least until he'd met that red-haired, money grubber at the meeting.

Collins warned his student that he would find himself boxed into a profit-oriented project, one that might not have any intellectual or scientific challenge. Five or ten years down the road he might be an administrator, manipulating budgets instead of molecules, far removed from the excitement of research. Is this what he had worked so hard for? Collins grew agitated at Daniel's lack of response, and finally tried to shock him into some sort of reaction by telling him he was selling out, leasing his brain to a company in return for a fancy salary and a nice place to live in the country.

But Daniel couldn't really see what was so wrong with a good salary and a nice house, especially after the crowded tenement life he had experienced for so many years. As the professor's warnings became more animated, Daniel's attention slipped farther away, to thoughts of diapers and bottles and happy children in the Connecticut countryside. It took his utmost concentration to pay attention to this man to whom he owed so much. Finally, Collins was out of arguments, and Daniel politely excused himself.

Even if Daniel had had any doubts about where his biochemical talents would take him they would have been dissipated once he saw the company research facility in Fairfax. It was, in short, an ideal place to work and an ideal place to live. It reminded him of the country scenes he had looked at in books as a child, and he knew that Eleanor and their children would love living there. So Daniel accepted the position at ACC, and he and Collins reached a sort of impasse, each accepting the other's choice, and vowing to keep in touch.

Daniel, Eleanor, and their firstborn took to Connecticut as if they had always been meant to live there. Daniel was assigned to study hormone function in several types of experimental animals, and found that his work was similar to what he had done in graduate school - with the major difference that he worked fewer hours for more pay. He actually had evenings and weekends now, to read and enjoy his wife and daughter.

Daniel was very pleased with his family's quick assimilation, because he at once saw that he had a great future with American Chemical. Here were the facilities to take his ideas, and farm them out to others so that they could be investigated faster than he could do so himself. Daniel was soon supervising others in carrying out projects that he had originated, acting as a manager although he was only a junior staff biochemist.

His creativity and ability to guide others did not go unnoticed by management. After 18 months, he had received a very generous raise and a promotion of not one, but two levels. As a unit manager, he now had a dozen biochemists under his direction, yet was free to pursue those projects that interested him the most. And although the company released junior-level scientists when the stock market crashed and the depression ensued, Daniel, with his ability to generate results, was not one of them.

The months passed and then the years, with Daniel rising in the company hierarchy as Eleanor furnished their new home, to which she added two more children. By 1935, Daniel was a branch manager, responsible for 48 endocrinologists, biochemists, and pharmacologists, and was emerging as a leader in the pharmaceutical component of the company. Daniel himself chose to focus on a pituitary fraction that seemed to regulate the ovarian cycle. Chemicals in this fraction would safely control a woman's ability to conceive.

It was a time of rapid growth for the industry, particularly in research and development. The advent of electrophoresis by Arne Wilhelm Tiselius meant that the complex protein fractions isolated from ground endocrine tissue could now be separated into their components. And Daniel, indeed nearly everyone in the research force at American, knew that it was just a matter of time until the body's own chemicals could be isolated, characterized, and put to work in medicine.

Being a division head, in charge of more than 100 scientists, was almost unheard of for a man in his forties. But Daniel was special in many ways. His ability to generate ideas faster than anyone could possibly test them out had grown over the years, as he educated himself in different fields by reading an impressive number of journals each week. Daniel was one of those rare scientists who could look at someone else's data, immediately see the holes in the work, and know what had to be done next. He could also bring together ideas from fields that, to anyone else, looked unrelated. This was why, for example, he would hire a botanist, a cell biologist, and an organic chemist to work on the same problem of manufacturing a certain drug. He wanted to see who could produce it the cheapest - the botanist who would extract it from a whole plant, the cell biologist who would try to grow only those cells that produced the drug, and the chemist, who would try to synthesize it in the lab.

But Daniel also rose up the corporate ladder simply because people liked him. His rather long gray hair and merry blue eyes, plus his springy step, had a way of communicating his excitement to all who worked with him. For the technicians, an encounter with Daniel always boosted their enthusiasm for their work, giving routine tasks a sense of overall purpose in the industry. No one who worked with or for Daniel ever forgot the experience.

By the 1960s, Daniel was appointed Scientific Director of American. Five divisions and 1200 employees reported to him. By 1970, Daniel had also become a very shrewd businessman. While his consultants explored new options in genetic engineering, and his safety experts kept the EPA and press off his back, he beefed up the Public Relations department, just in case something unpleasant became publicly known. He instituted a monthly newsletter that made American look like a wonderfully safe place to work, and issued frequent press bulletins that highlighted products and profits, but never mentioned how the facility dealt with its wastes. Always popular with his workers and the press, Daniel began to look even more like the beloved head of one big happy corporate family.

Until the mercury problem.

It had started in 1978 when several mothers in the area tried to nurse their newborns and couldn't - the infants balked at nature's food. When an observant pediatrician noticed that five patients in one week had reported the same problem, she had collected milk samples from the mothers and had them analyzed in a chemistry laboratory at the Yale University School of Medicine.

The milk was found to contain .05 micrograms per milliliter of methyl mercury; one hundred times higher than the allowable level in drinking water. And there were also traces of cadmium. All of the women lived within three blocks of each other, in the Sunny Oaks subdivision located a mile downstream from the affluent running Daniel's plant. And both methyl mercury and cadmium had been found in the wells supplying their homes. Daniel had gotten his safety department onto the problem immediately.

But they had not been fast enough for Joan Archmont. No sooner could you say "methyl mercury" than Archmont had dug up a pathetic picture of a woman holding her teenaged daughter, a victim of Minimata disease. The young woman had been profoundly mentally retarded and physically deformed since birth, because her mother, who had suffered no ill- effects, had eaten fish contaminated with mercury during her pregnancy. The mercury had concentrated in the woman's body, and had concentrated further in the brain, nerves, and red blood cells of her unborn child, where it did extensive damage.

The people of Fairfax did not soon forget the image of the young woman, although they couldn't have even if they had tried. Archmont continued to give weekly updates on the Fairfax county spontaneous abortion rate for weeks following the detection of the chemical in breast milk. She also did an unforgettable segment on cadmium poisoning, linking it to kidney and lung failure. The tendency of cadmium to accumulate in vegetables and grains sent many a home gardener out to the family plot with a hoe.

Joan Archmont carefully planned her reports, guiding the viewers' thinking in ways that they could not usually detect. She typically led off by presenting accepted scientific evidence, and followed up with reports of what was flowing out of the American plant. She never overtly stated a causal link between the two - she left that to her viewers, who were even more inclined to tune in again when they thought that they were coming to a brilliant medical conclusion all on their own.

Not surprisingly, the ratings soared - at American's expense. And when a leak of toxic metals was actually discovered in the plant and quickly corrected, the image of the do-good chemical company on the hill had been irreparably tarnished. And Daniel's with it.

All that had been two years ago. And now old Joan was at it again full force, parading around the Down's kids and headache sufferers. Daniel sat in her outer office the morning after the broadcast about Jason. After 10 minutes of leafing through a People magazine and feeling as if he were slipping into a coma, the reporter finally appeared, and motioned him into her inner office. Joan Archmont was probably the only person in the world who thought herself important enough to keep Daniel Weil, Chairman of the Board of the American Chemical Company, waiting. He said as much.

"Thanks for the compliment. I trust you saw last night's broadcast?" inquired the reporter with mock innocence.

"Me and the rest of the county, I'm sure. Let's just hope the national press doesn't pick it up."

"On the contrary, I hope it does. CBS in New York is on the line with my assistant. It's a damn good story, don't you think?"

The woman's condescending attitude was driving Daniel to the first thoughts of murder he had ever entertained. He was glad that he didn't have high blood pressure.

"Actually, no. Have you ever heard the phrases 'case-control', 'sample size', or 'double blind'? Perhaps not - one can't expect a reporter to have heard of, let alone understand, the nuances of the scientific method."

"Mr. Weil."

"That's Dr. Weil, Ms. Archmont."

"Dr. Weil, Chairman, Sir, our viewers don't care about scientific mumbo jumbo. They want the straight story. And that's exactly what I give them."

"Well, I'll agree that you're certainly giving them something, but it comes from the wrong end of the horse. Do you really think that you can parade around sick children and throw around numbers and chemical formulas without explaining anything, without putting it into some balanced perspective? I guess they just don't teach that in journalism school. Ratings above truth, and all that."

Joan was silent for a moment, and looked as if she was deciding whether or not to say something. Apparently she decided in the affirmative.

"Dr. Weil, we're getting nowhere hurling insults at one another. I asked you to come here today because I thought it only fair to inform you about the content of my broadcast tomorrow night."

"What else could you possibly say? Are you going to take all the women with uncombable hair or kids with zits and blame it on us? What about drug abuse - that would be a new angle."

"Please, Dr. Weil. I'm quite serious."

"Okay. Go on."

"You remember the methyl mercury situation two years ago, right? At the time, I thought it might be wise to investigate your personal background a bit, just in case something truly catastrophic happened someday at the plant. You are a beacon among industrialists, and I thought some personal background information might come in handy someday." "And what sordid little things did you find?"

"Nothing sordid at all. In fact, I uncovered a past that should make you proud."

"I'm afraid I don't understand the connection of my past to the current situation."

"You will. I dug way back, first talking to scientists who had gone to grad school with you, and then to some friends from your childhood. Does the name Micah Lefkowitz ring a bell?"

Daniel sat deep in thought for a moment or two. Sixty-odd years was a long way to think back. But he did remember Micah, a friend from his boyhood who had often accompanied him to the Settlement House library.

"Yes, I do remember him vaguely. But how did you get in touch with him? What is he doing?"

"I had a journalism intern do my sleuthing. She hunted around the stores of the Lower East Side that are run today by the grandchildren of the people who ran them back when you were a boy. That's how we found Micah, who is still there running a dress shop, although his family lives out on Long Island. He was only too happy to talk about you."

"But why didn't he contact me?"

"He claimed that he tried several times, after he'd read about your rise at American. But he never got an answer."

That much could easily be true. Daniel hardly ever looked at his mail, particularly not the personal letters. That's what secretaries were for.

"Anyway, Micah told my assistant some very interesting things about your mother."

"My mother was a wonderful woman," Daniel shouted angrily.

"Indeed she was. In fact, we learned that she was instrumental in gaining reforms for the shirtwaist industry. In particular, reforms in the area of worker safety."

"I don't seem to recall that."

"You were only eight years old at the time, but your mother, along with 20,000 other garment workers, went on strike in 1909 to demand safer working conditions. And after the tragic Triangle Shirtwaist fire in 1911, she went on to organize the women on Rivington Street to demand further reforms - and of course, after that disaster their demands were heard."

Daniel had turned ashen. He was incapable of speech. All at once the horror of what he had witnessed as a child, until then deeply buried in his subconscious, came spilling into his awareness. He could picture almost as if it were happening now; the women screaming as they leapt from the blazing windows, the young man and woman holding hands as they jumped, and the smacking sound of their bodies hitting the pavement, then the thuds of others landing on top of them.

And when the initial horror of remembrance passed, he saw what the ruthless reporter was getting at. The terrible irony of what his mother, a factory worker, had done to champion safety, contrasted with what he, a powerful industrialist, could not be bothered to do.

He would be characterized as no better than the owner of the shirtwaist factory who had ignored the pleas to rebuild his wooden structure in 1909, only to be responsible for nearly 200 deaths just two years later.

Daniel was furious. Since conversation was not possible and violence was, he guiltily left the lair of Joan Archmont.

He walked in a trance to his next appointment at the local hospital, where he was to have a routine physical examination. He would have forgotten it in his distress but for the nagging cough that seemed to intensify when he was angry. Both the cough and his anger were happening more and more frequently lately, no thanks to Joan Archmont, and he was quite sure that his physician would recommend tranquilizers, a vacation, or perhaps even a psychiatrist to get at the source of his anxiety.

But he had not in the least expected what actually happened.

He had LUNG CANCER!

But he simply COULD NOT have lung cancer. He didn't smoke, had never smoked. Surely the spot on the chest x-ray was a mistake. They had gotten his plates mixed up with someone else's. Or maybe if they really were his, he had a cyst or other benign growth.

People who didn't smoke just didn't get lung cancer.

But later that day, his doctor compassionately explained that people who didn't smoke sometimes did get lung cancer, often a type called an adenocarcinoma. To be sure that Daniel indeed had this condition, other tests would be necessary. And of course there was the Federal Cancer Institute. He knew

Institute. He knew Jacob Poldosky, the former director of FCI, and, through several of his scientists, he had met a Dr. Musso. They owed him one for supplying that platinum analog last year, and the methotrexate derivative the year before. He'd call tomorrow morning and get himself immediately into the most promising FCI clinical trial, even if it meant a short stay in Washington.

Daniel lay back on the pillows, his hands on his chest, and relaxed a bit. No tumor was going to claim someone with his abundant resources. He sighed and turned on the TV.

And there, her plasticine face glowing with satisfaction, was the triumphant Joan Archmont.

CHAPTER 5

THE COMMITMENT

January 20, 1959

The score was 64 all; it was the semi-finals of the sub- state tournament in Springfield, Missouri. The coaches, the players, and the crowd knew THIS WAS IT. The Culverton High School Tigers had played their best season in a decade. They were 18-2 and both losses had occurred in a two-game stretch when Robert Gordon and Joe Hardwell had been out with the flu. They were, by consensus, the best class B team in the state, except possibly for their opponents, the Lebanon Mavericks, who had gone undefeated for the year.

The sportswriters were there, the college coaches were there, and each school could have filled the stands alone. After a tension-packed time-out, Robert Gordon stepped to the foul line. Four seconds were left and this was the second overtime. The teams had played absolutely dead even; this was the moment of truth.

Seven thousand enthusiasts were dead silent. Robert bounced the ball four times, his trademark, then released it with a classic motion, a smooth release allowing him to lead the Tri-County league in shooting percentage. The ball looked short, but almost as if it had a life of its own, it leaped over the front edge of the rim, and dropped softly through the net.

The noise was deafening. All 7000 fans, it seemed, were on their feet, screaming. And for the first time in a long game, and an even longer season, Robert heard the crowd. Usually he was aware only of the players, coaches, and referees. But tonight was special. He drank in every human response, even the inane yells of the cheerleaders. He felt a surge of excitement. His adrenaline was flowing and the rush from being the center of the crowd's attention was palpable. He took his patented four bounces, and let fly again. This one dropped through with ease, and the Tigers were up by two. The Tiger coaches were screaming for the team to settle down, and come up the court with a full defensive press - but, no fouls!

The four seconds seemed like a lifetime to Robert. As was always the case, he picked up the best shooter for the other team. The ball was being brought up rapidly, and Robert was staying between his man, an all-state guard for the Mavericks, and the goal. The boy took the out-of-bounds pass at mid-court, feinted left, and moved quickly right. He had a step on Robert, but Robert knew him well, and knew his major fault. He couldn't shoot without glancing at the basket first. The boy drove the right sideline, and Robert, a quarter-step behind, caught the glance at the basket. Stevenson left the floor with his "big college" jump shot, but Robert had gone up at the glance. The ball left Stevenson's hand, only to be slapped away dramatically by Robert's outstretched fingers. The horn sounded, and absolute pandemonium broke loose. The frenzied crowd flooded onto the court, enveloping the ecstatic team.

To Robert, the Culverton High School Tigers were his family. They had lost in sub-state two years in a row; Robert and Joe had been all-conference and had lead this team since they were sophomores. Finally, at last, they would go to the state tournament and play the best from across the state. What an unforgettable night!

Robert awoke with a start. It was really 1963. The dream always ended with him bolting upright in bed, almost as thrilled as he had been on that night when it really happened. Even though it regularly tore him from sleep, the memory of the big game was a great comfort to Robert, especially now, when he was so dissatisfied with his life.

He wasn't quite sure just why he was unhappy. He supposed he should be grateful that he had landed a job so easily, fresh out of college. He was a chemical engineer for the International Minerals and Chemical Corporation (IMCC), doing well at work, and making enough money to enjoy an evening out now and then. He had lots of friends, and he had no trouble getting dates. Whatever it was about his blond hair and blue-eyed all-American looks that had attracted the girls in high school was still at work.

But something was missing. Certainly he couldn't continue in this pattern of hard-to define boredom for his whole life. Oh, how he yearned for the days when a basketball game was all he needed for that elusive feeling of complete contentment. The total commitment of driving to the basket with no concern for the consequences; the elation of the just-right pass; the adrenaline of the last-second shot. God, how he had loved it.

In fact, senior year of high school was the happiest time that Robert could remember - maybe that was why it replayed itself in his dreams so often, even now, after college. High school was when his family had finally settled in one place for longer than a year or two. And there were certainly worse places to spend one's adolescence than Culverton, Missouri. It was surely better than Poker, Wyoming, where he had been born in 1941. He and World War II had debuted at about the same time.

Robert's father had been exempted from military service because of his domestic value as a locomotive engineer. In most families this would have been regarded as a blessing, but Robert often wished that his father had gone overseas. He had many negative memories of the man. His father had a sharp mind, but had never gotten beyond the fifth grade, a fact that he seemed to hold against everyone he knew, particularly his family. He was universally dissatisfied with life, and gradually turned to alcohol for solace. Robert would never forget the screaming drunken rages that became an expected, but never understood, part of his childhood. His tardiness and increasingly poor work performance at the railroad were a constant economic threat to the family. They moved often, from town to town first in Wyoming, then to Washington State, California and finally Missouri.

The Florida apartment was hot and muggy, even at 3 in the morning. Robert rose and lit a cigarette, then walked over to the bay window overlooking the beach. He didn't like working at IMCC, but he did love the beach. The sound of the waves was somehow reassuring, always coming in, never stopping for anything or anybody. It reminded him of the rhythmic pounding of his feet on the track during meets in high school, when Robert had been a top miler. Half asleep, he wondered if the rhythm of the waves on the ocean and pounding feet on a track had the same physiological effect on the body, somehow releasing a comforting hormone that made stress momentarily vanish. A run on the beach would be nice now; but he was just too tired.

Robert crushed out his cigarette, thinking about the recent publicity that smoking was unhealthy. Should he believe the billboards and TV ads with their athletic young people puffing happily away, or the scattered medical reports linking smoking to disease? The cigarette and lung cancer link in particular had him worried. Cancer sounded like such a terrible way to go. But at the same time, he admitted to himself that he really enjoyed smoking. It gave him a certain release from the inexplicable inner tension that he constantly felt.

Robert sank into his beaten up easy chair and started to drift off to sleep. On the edge of consciousness, he remembered falling asleep in the hospital wards in Kansas City, where his mother worked as a nurse. Babysitters were hard to find back then, and it was not unusual for Robert to find himself sleeping on a hospital gurney, not far from the nursing station, his mother the charge nurse. Lena Gordon was a superb nurse, and an outstanding organizer, a person the hospital administration depended upon to get the job done, whatever it might be. And in the crazy world of a hospital, almost anything could come up. Staffing was always short, and babysitters for active young boys scarce. As a result, the rules were bent a little for Nurse Gordon's son, and Robert dozed on in the hospital hallway. It happened often.

He could almost smell the old Kansas City Research Hospital, where the antiseptic odors mingled with the unmistakable odors of illness and despair, just by thinking about the place. He remembered the quiet times of sleep interrupted by the clanging of bells and the furious activity when a clinical "event" occurred. Then the nurses and physicians would rush into a room to try to prevent the inevitable death of a patient suffering a heart attack. Those people in white seemed so competent, so in control, so qualified. Yet Robert learned early on that despite these efforts, the patient usually died. How frustrating it must be to have someone's life literally in your hands, and to lose it!

By 4:00 a.m., Robert slipped into bed and fell back to sleep. He had a dream that was to change his life. He would later wonder why it had taken so very long for him to have that dream. In the dream, Robert wasn't in the white laboratory coat of the chemical engineer, nor did he have his slide rule and charts. He wasn't solving an intricate problem in fluid flow dynamics. Instead, he saw himself with a stethoscope and a white jacket in a brightly-colored room with a patient. He felt the frustration, the despair, the longing and the pain of the elderly woman, who had such faith in him. A frail hand reached out and a weak voice trembled, "Doctor, can you help me?" As he touched the woman, stroking her arm to comfort her, he felt a sense of life-force flowing from him to her. Suddenly, her face seemed more alive, her color better, and her voice stronger, just from his touch. "Doctor, please do everything you can to help me. I want to stay around this world longer. There is so much to do."

Robert, the physician, left the room. His dream was becoming fuzzy. He felt some satisfaction because he had comforted the old woman, but he couldn't help but wonder about her sense of self-preservation and will to live, after 80 some years of what he assumed had been a healthy and productive life. He wondered what it must be like to be old and sick.

A clanging went off in his head, and Robert looked around. Was it a "code blue?" As he awakened he reached out and knocked his alarm clock off the bedside table and realized where he was. No, he wasn't a doctor. It was just his alarm telling him it was time to go to work. Back to IMCC and the life of a chemical engineer.

Robert dragged himself from the lumpy bed, more tired than usual because of his 3:00 a.m. bout with insomnia. He was aware of the unpleasant odor and taste of last night's cigarettes and beer. He looked about his messy, drab apartment and understood a little the frustration of the old woman in his dream. Like her, he wanted to live, wanted to go on, but he knew that he was not headed in the right direction.

Within two weeks of the dream, Robert had made his decision.

He had understood the calling. He was meant to be a doctor, and had in fact been preparing for this, although he didn't realize it, since his childhood days in the hospital ward. Chemical engineering wasn't right for him. The Sputnik mentality and the fear of a nation over the lack of engineering skills had pushed many a high school senior into selecting engineering and technical careers for which they were not well suited. He had been one of them.

Robert was an excellent student. In college he made A's and B's in physics, calculus, and fluid dynamics even with fraternities, beer, and girls occupying a major part of his time. A little study the night before an exam was really all that he ever had to do. The only courses he really enjoyed and were challenged by were those in the biological sciences. He had found chemistry, biology and zoology far more stimulating than his engineering courses.

He knew now that he had made the wrong career choice. His commitment was clear and he felt overwhelming relief when his decision was finally made.

He was going back to school. Medical school.

Mary Margaret was back home in Tennessee. It was 1963, and she was wondering just what she would do next. Her father, a Presbyterian minister, wanted her to go back to school, perhaps to get involved in the social sciences and in some way help other people. Her mother, who had a strong social presence in the community, preferred marriage for her daughter, and a marriage of some stature. She already had one or two good candidates lined up, although neither they nor Mary Margaret knew it - young men from prominent local families. But Mary Margaret wasn't at all sure of her own feelings. Two years in a girl's school in Missouri and now back home. She really didn't feel comfortable with her status as a part-time student and a part-time member of the Harding family, and her thoughts kept going back to St. Louis. And to a certain young man.

God, she really missed him. It was funny how you could spend the better part of two years with a person, memorizing every facial feature, every nuance of behavior, every personality quirk, and then when you are apart, have trouble conjuring up what he even vaguely looked like.

She and Robert had enjoyed their time together, but had not thought much about the future. Now she found that she felt more for him than she had thought possible. Maybe the separation had been good, at least in terms of straightening out her own feelings. She knew now that she loved him, and had since their first date. But at the same time, she knew that there was some basic problem in their relationship, some hard-to-define deficiency. It's not that they didn't care for one another, nor that they didn't have fun together. Rather, Robert couldn't seem to focus properly. Back in college he had sometimes seemed unhappy, not completely listening to what she was saying, and she couldn't tell whether it was something about her or not. He had finished his engineering degree with honors in the top five percent of his class, but it had apparently come so easily to him that he wasn't even proud or excited about his success.

And if his academic marks were high, his social marks were just the opposite. It was almost as if he was destined to repeat the mistakes of his father, a man they rarely discussed. Robert found himself in a pattern of getting through school during the day, and drinking beer every night, keeping himself too busy to think much about what he was doing or why he was doing it. Like his father, Robert was suffering from a basic dissatisfaction with the way his life was going. And although he and Mary Margaret had spent many evenings together, he could never completely open up to her, tell her what was bothering him. So she wondered what was wrong, and sometimes didn't hear from him for days at a time. As a result, she was never really sure of him, even when they were "lavelered". So she never allowed herself to think much about any kind of a future with him. And now, nearly one year after their graduation, she rarely heard from Robert. She wasn't really surprised. Maybe she was the reason for his distance.

About three months ago she had received a rare letter from him. In it, she again sensed his frustration. And to her relief, it seemed to stem from his career, not her. His letter had mentioned the ins and outs of his job at IMCC, descriptions of his friends (she skipped over mention of the female ones), and of his drab apartment with the spectacular view of the ocean. But what struck her was the last paragraph of the letter, which she still couldn't quite figure out. She'd memorized it after the third reading, not daring to put into words what it had made her hope.

Mary Margaret, I find myself thinking of you often. No, more than often. I miss our times together. I guess what I'm saying is that I miss you. I've an idea. Since you don't have a full-time position in Tennessee, why don't you come down here to Florida and join me? You could find a job here, and we could be together. I miss you so.

Robert

Mary Margaret didn't know what to make of the letter. Was he lonely and homesick? Was he unable to make the leap from college to the real world? Or did he really miss her? Before she left the comfort of her parents' home, she had to know more about what Robert truly wanted, even if he didn't yet know himself.

So she had waited a few days, then written back to Robert that he really needed to clarify his feelings for her before they should resume a relationship. She'd taken a chance, she knew, and when she'd heard nothing further from him, she feared that she had lost him. He'd just find someone down there. After all, he'd never had any trouble finding female friends.

Now, three months after she had received Robert's letter, Mary Margaret was lazing about at home, her parents at the usual Sunday afternoon church social hour, which often stretched into the evening. She was soaking up the sun on the veranda, and as usual, all she could think about was how her letter must have turned Robert off, of how stupid she'd been to lose him. Maybe she should have gone to Florida, taken whatever developed. Maybe she should call him.

Just then, the phone rang, startling her out of her reverie. She ran into the kitchen to answer it, a little lightheaded from lying in the sun. And when she said hello, for a second she didn't believe who was on the other end.

"M M? (His pet name for her.) Is that you? This is Robert."

"Oh my. Robert, I was just lying here thinking about you. About us."

"M M, I miss you, and I love you. I think about you all the time," blurted Robert.

Mary Margaret was shocked into silence for a moment or two, then composed herself and said, in a shaking voice, "Robert, I can't come to Florida, it just won't work."

Now there was a silence on the other end, and her heart stopped. Was he going to behave erratically, shout at her? Hang up the phone? She had experienced all of these with him and nothing would surprise her. But what came next certainly did surprise her.

"Mary Margaret, will you marry me? Will you marry me right now? I need you," Robert asked quickly, in a firm and sure voice.

Mary Margaret nearly dropped the receiver. Of all the things that he could have said, she had least expected this. Her mind was a jumble, but somehow she heard herself answer without hesitation, "Yes, yes, of course. Oh Robert, I love you so much."

Robert was standing in line. He and about 60 other St. Louis University medical students were in the middle of an anatomy practical exam. Various anatomical parts dissected from their cadavers were laid out on a table, with small pins with numbers in them. The exercise was to identify the muscle, nerve, artery, or other structure impaled by the numbered pin. It reminded Robert of a game of pin the tail on the donkey, with somewhat higher stakes.

Each student trooped slowly through the maze of disembodied human parts, writing in a blue examination booklet furtively so that others could not copy the answers. Robert kept a watchful eye on Barry Monder. Good old Barry pretended to be everyone's pal, but then when your back was turned, he'd switch the pins on the parts so that the students behind him would write down wrong answers. This, of course, would help Barry's own class standing, something of vital importance in these days before the "pass-fail" revolution in medical schools.

Dishonest behavior was not all that unusual in the highly competitive world of medical school. Robert had even seen students pour coke or spit into other students' experiments in the lab. And Barry was one of the worst offenders. Great standards for a physician, Robert thought. But honesty and integrity weren't all that important to the professors charged with molding the young doctors-in- training. Like the four years of college that had funnelled these top-notch students into medical school, grades seemed to be all that mattered. And it didn't matter how you got them.

The anatomy lab was hot, the formaldehyde odor of the preserved human tissues overwhelming, and the pressure to succeed great. The atmosphere would sicken most people, but Robert thrived in it. He knew all of the structures in the exam, and had fun whizzing through them, Barry Monder or no Barry Monder.

In the hallway after the exam, Robert stopped to talk with Susan Amber. Susan was not only a bright young woman, ranking in the top 5 of the class, but she was also a very attractive woman. Her shimmering long red hair and ample figure made her instantly stand out from the white-clad crowd, even when she had it all tucked away as best she could. And Susan did seem to downplay her looks. She felt they were a disadvantage. She had to go out of her way to prove that she was just as smart, if not smarter, than one of the prep school scholars in the class. She had once told Robert that she was never sure whether people, especially men, were interested in her or her appearance. Robert had actually wondered the same thing about himself at times, but no one had ever questioned his intelligence because of his appearance.

Robert and Susan shared a love of anatomy, physiology and biochemistry, and worked well together in the library and in the laboratory. The harsh competitive shell that many of the students erected around themselves wasn't there between Robert and Susan, and they were free to explore the intellectual challenges of the study of medicine. They were good friends.

"Susan, what did you think of the anatomy test?" asked Robert.

"About average, I'd say. I'm glad we studied so hard, though. At least the problems were rather straightforward. I did okay - you must've too."

"Yeah, I did okay. It helps having someone to work with. Thank you."

"Did Barry move any pins today?"

"No, but I was watching, and I think he knew it."

"I really can't even stand to be in the same room with the guy. Someone should pin a tail on him," Susan retorted, with more venom than Robert was used to hearing in her voice.

"Hey, what's the matter?"

"Oh, he just gets to me. Calls me 'honey' or 'sweetie' all the time, acts as if I don't deserve to be here. I bet he doesn't call you his little sweetie. He makes me sick."

Robert was unnerved and attempted to change the direction of the conversation. "What did you think of Shanklin's lecture on the biochemistry and immunology of cancer cells?"

But the lecture that had electrified him had the opposite effect on his friend. Her face clouded as she shuffled her books and glanced at her watch. "Shanklin is a great lecturer, and I really enjoyed it intellectually." She was silent, and seemed even more disturbed.

"What's wrong, Susan?" Robert asked in a concerned, gentle voice.

Tears spurted. "My mother died last summer from breast cancer. It's been a difficult year for me, and the problem of cancer causes such emotional turmoil that I am having some difficulty concentrating on malignancy as just another medical school topic. I mean, it's such a personal thing to me. I just can't look at it as an objective physician. Only as a grieving daughter."

Robert thought for a moment, trying to formulate a helpful but sensitive answer.

"In time you will. And maybe this experience, although it must have been horrible, will give you a unique perspective so that you may someday be able to offer some comfort to patients like your mother," he said with more conviction than he actually felt. Robert was fascinated by the odd behavior of cancer cells, but had no experience with people whose lives were threatened by those cells, as Susan had. He thought some of the very skinny and weak patients he had seen as a child being carted around the hospital where his mother worked might have had cancer, but he couldn't recall every hearing the word "cancer" back then.

"Thanks, Robert. You're always such a comfort to me." She squeezed his arm and then took off for her next class.

Susan had hit upon something that Robert had been thinking about lately. The cancer problem. There seemed to be two sides to it. The exciting laboratory aspect of investigating just what those crazed cells did, and the hope that someday research might lead to better treatment or a cure. And then there was the tremendous emotional problems of the patient. How did such a person deal with the knowledge that certain death would come soon? How did a patient get the most out of the time left? Robert wondered how he'd deal with the problem when it came time to take care of patients next year. He knew he was unusually skilled in the lab, and could pass any exam with just a few hours of study. But could he handle real people, sick people? After all, that was the real test, the important test, of being a doctor. That was what was in his dream. But for the first time in his life, he wondered about his own ability.

It was 8:05 a.m. and rounds were late in starting. The "roundsmen" were ready - the chief resident, the assistant chief resident, the senior residents, and the junior residents, all gathered on ward 4-B. Robert was a mere junior medical student, the bottom of the heap.

Professor Joseph Xavier was now eight minutes late. Patients weren't the only ones kept waiting in a hospital, Robert thought. But of course, this was the academic side of things. One waited for at least five minutes for an assistant professor, ten to fifteen minutes for an associate professor, and forever, if necessary, for a full professor.

Robert's legs ached. He had spent the previous day engaged in a high honor - holding the liver aside for one of the school's great surgeons during major stomach surgery. Four hours of holding a liver in one position. The technical aspects interested him, given his mechanical ability with automobiles and other machinery, but he knew he would never be a surgeon. His legs simply wouldn't stand it. Robert played basketball two nights a week, and ran four to five days each week, so his legs were good and strong. But athletics involved movement. Surgery was another matter. He had no interest in standing still for hours in a surgical suite, even if it meant he could become intimately acquainted with a liver.

He was also bored by standing at ward 4-B, waiting for professor Joseph Xavier to make his grand entrance. The man was a great academician and the author of over 100 papers on renal physiology. Robert was appropriately impressed and even intimidated by the professor's academic credentials, but he disliked him as a human being. Xavier's rounds were always characterized by the one-upmanship of having read the latest journal first, or having written the latest paper. And being on a paper of course wasn't good enough - you had to be the first author to attract his attention.

But by far the most offensive aspect of making rounds with Xavier was his description of patients as "cases". Robert vowed that he would never use this word in discussing patients. It seemed to Robert that as one trained and graduated from a medical student to a lowly intern to a resident and then eventually a great professor, the patient became more and more remote, more of a "case". Less and less an individual. Robert just couldn't comprehend this - for him things were just the opposite. The more he learned about the patient and disease, the higher his regard became for the person within each patient.

Suddenly, the huffing and puffing of professor Xavier's labored breathing (caused by 40-odd years of heavy smoking, Robert thought) could be heard, and he appeared from around the corner, charging down the corridor toward the nurse's station.

"Well, it's a beautiful day out, and I want to finish rounds by 10:00. I have a medical grand rounds to give at 3:00 p.m.," he announced as if he was to deliver a Nobel lecture. Such a great man, the almighty professor, Robert thought as he saw one of the interns already taking notes, not wanting to miss a syllable of what the man uttered. And so Xavier and his entourage of admiring young physicians went off on rounds, and discussed the five "interesting cases".

The first, who had acute glomerulonephritis, illustrated the principles of kidney function; the second, who was two days post-myocardial infarction, taught the students how to deal with the aftermath of a heart attack; the third demonstrated the damage of a severe bacterial infection in the bloodstream. Then there was Mrs. Turnkey, who was a beautiful exhibition of surgical complications. She had recently undergone a routine gallbladder removal, and had developed bowel obstruction and inflammation throughout the lining of her intestine. She was on intravenous nutrition and was in tremendous pain and discomfort, requiring multiple medications and antibiotics. Professor Xavier really enjoyed going over the complexity of that case. But all Robert could see was a suffering patient.

Finally, there was Thomas Averhouse. Thomas, at 34, was not much older than Robert. He had a poorly characterized cancer in his lungs, liver and bones. The tumors had shrunk a bit from chemotherapy, but they were now growing again. It was curious that Thomas had been included as a "case" for rounds. The students, interns and residents seldom discussed the cancer patients on the medical ward. These patients were usually put at the ends of the hallways and were cared for by the interns. Not much "teaching content". Thomas was an exception, probably because of his age and the fact that he had responded to chemotherapy, which was a relatively new way of treating cancer in the late 1960s. Even given the interest in Thomas' situation, rounds only stopped there for about five minutes, and no discussion ensued on what might be done in the future to deal with his progressive malignancy.

It was 1968, and Robert felt good, as anyone would who was about to graduate from medical school. His grades had been high, his concentration admirable, his married life happy, and he and Mary Margaret had a son. Mary Margaret had worked to support them throughout medical school in various office jobs. Without her help, and without low interest government loans, Robert knew that he would never have been able to go to medical school. He was now a senior and would very soon be an intern and then a resident, and would finally earn a little money. He could plan their future!

The family finances were helped by the fact that Robert's talents extended beyond chemical engineering and medicine. While in medical school, he had used his skill in cards to earn a substantial income from his more well-endowed and less talented classmates. Poker contributed to the Gordon family income at a level on a par with government loans and Mary Margaret's jobs. But despite this additional source of income, the Gordons were finishing medical school over $50,000 in debt. Robert looked forward to his upcoming internship, at a salary of about $10,000 per year.

Graduation was a month away, and Robert had just returned from Boston, where he had spent two months externing on the cancer wards at the Chronic Diseases Hospital (CDH). This had been a most rewarding experience, one that was to profoundly influence the young doctor's future.

Many of the cancer patients at CDH had been shipped over from Harvard and Peter Bent Bringham. This seemed to be in line with Robert's previous experience at St. Louis University, where the "interesting cases" were retained on the teaching service and the less interesting cases - the cancer patients -

were shuttled elsewhere. As an extern at CDH, Robert had complete responsibility for the care of these unwanted but to him, special patients. And they were too ill to care, or even realize, that their "doctor" had not yet completed medical school. But Robert seemed to have his own brand of kindness and caring that quickly endeared him to the patients. The smiles on their faces when he entered their rooms assured him that he had made the right decision in becoming a physician.

But Robert wasn't the only one in the medical profession who felt drawn to people who had cancer. In Missouri and then in Boston, Robert met two physicians who called themselves oncologists. He was intrigued by their conviction that cancer could be beaten. They were giving various drugs to their patients, in an attempt to induce a remission - not just wait for the inevitable to occur. They were actually doing something!

Since the turn of the century it had been well established that surgery and radiation treatment were occasionally effective in controlling and sometimes even curing a local or regional cancer. Lymphoma, a cancer of the lymph nodes, had yielded some to highly toxic chemicals given to halt the rapidly dividing cancer cells. Robert's experiences under the oncologists taught him that there was a wide variety of toxic chemicals, under the general category of chemotherapy, which could induce remissions in selected patients with cancer. It was clear to him that these oncologists were part of a wave of the future. Physicians could and someday would routinely use systemic chemical therapy to reduce the cancer cell load or maybe even cure the disease, at least in some people.

The attitude of this new breed of doctor, the medical oncologist, was in striking contrast to the other professors at St. Louis University and the Boston hospitals. Most were of the opinion that there was no effective treatment for metastatic cancer. Attempts at treatment, especially using chemicals, were regarded as foolhardy. It was 1968.

By the time he graduated from medical school, Dr. Robert Gordon had learned several important lessons. One was that breaking new ground in medicine required a continuing acquisition of information and laboratory capability. Secondly, one must not believe too strongly the words of the great professors. Too often, he had learned, they were merely parroting what they had heard from their professors and were not a source of new knowledge. Robert preferred to listen to younger physicians who had fresh and novel ideas. Thirdly, Robert had decided that he had to devote himself to one area of medicine. His love for biochemistry, physiology and immunology and his clinical experiences on the cancer wards and his natural compassion for human suffering had made this decision, unlike his push into chemical engineering, an easy one - and the right one.

He was going to become a cancer specialist, a medical oncologist.

Robert interned at Barnes Hospital in St. Louis. It was a hell of an experience for a fledgling physician. There were too few interns, too many patients, and too much illness for the job to be done well. The interns worked 18 hours a day, taking care of patients who were critically ill and in need of professional assistance beyond the skills of someone fresh out of medical school. The residents were a great help, when they could be found. Robert learned early; the system was set up to serve the doctor more than the patient. Senior physicians were only available by phone after 5:00 p.m. And the expertise of the professors could hardly be counted on. They came in for rounds and were of no use at all in the middle of the night, when the patients typically would fall apart.

Robert was up on his knees repetitively pounding the chest of a 68-year-old man who had gone into cardiac arrest. The man's heart muscle was so weakened that it could no longer adequately supply blood to the rest of the body. The compromised blood supply had further lowered his oxygen carrying capacity, and the man suffered from an abnormal heart rhythm, the deadly ventricular fibrillation. By repetitive cardiac compression and electrical shock, Robert and his team were attempting to revive the patient.

In the midst of this emergency, a nurse came to the door and beckoned to Robert.

"Dr. Gordon, you have a telephone call," she said, as if he was just sitting at his desk gazing out the window, not desperately hammering at a dying man's chest.

"Goddammit, Nurse Sheldon," Robert gasped, "can't you see that we are in the middle of a resuscitation? Take the number and tell them I'll call back." He continued to pound on his patient's chest.

Nurse Sheldon was a royal pain in the ass. She always seemed to have three items of dubious urgency to tell him over the phone at 3:00 a.m., when he had just fallen asleep. Two of those pieces of information were totally inconsequential, a patient who needed a laxative and another who wanted a sleeping pill, for example. However, Robert had developed the skill of waking to full alertness instantaneously, because her third report was always serious - a patient was in shock, in cardiac arrest, or had just pulled out three of the tubes that were supporting life. She had the curious inability to distinguish these facts in terms of importance, and the alertness of the intern unfortunate enough to be the recipient of her phone call was the only thing standing between life and death for that one unlucky patient in three who truly needed help. And unfortunately, the nurse seemed to have taken a liking to Robert.

In spite of Nurse Sheldon's interruption, his patient survived. As Robert walked back to the nurse's station, he was relieved that the man's life had been saved, but at the same time he was saddened, because he knew that most of these resuscitations were only useful in the short term. The patients usually arrested again, and ultimately died, if they had the kind of severe heart disease that had lead to the initial cardiac event. But such was the purpose of the intern: be there and do what you could for the short term, and hope that the longer term problem would take care of itself.

Robert picked up the telephone at the nurse's station. While he waited for an answer, he noticed the chaos around him. The nurse's station looked more like a garbage dump than the hub of the fourth floor of a large hospital. The mess reflected the long and arduous night. Three patients had died, two had bled massively, and three additional patients had been resuscitated. The stench of rotting blood and feces was everywhere and even the disinfectants were unable to suppress it. Paper was strewn all about as the nurses worked through the night, short-staffed and unable to maintain and file records simultaneously.

The voice on the other end of the phone was so hysterical that at first Robert didn't recognize it. Then he became alarmed.

"Robert! Robert! The mail just came in! I'm so excited!"

"Hold on, what happened? Did we win a sweepstakes?"

"Not we, you! You have been accepted!"

"Wait, M M, slow down. Tell me what you're babbling about," Robert asked calmly, although his insides were beginning to churn with expectancy. Could this be what he had been waiting for?

"You have just been accepted as a clinical associate at the Federal Cancer Institute. On the medicine branch, with Dr. Adrian Free. It's just what you wanted!"

Robert couldn't believe it. He felt his spirits soar. It indeed was just what he wanted, just what he had hoped for, what he dreamed of.

To an aspiring oncologist, "mecca" was the FCI. He knew that his peers were fighting like cats and dogs to get into these research programs. And for several reasons. Many young physicians were truly dedicated to the idea of research and wanted to become more adept in their profession. It was 1970. Others simply, and understandably, wanted to avoid Vietnam.

As in any high pressure situation, people used both their capabilities and their influence to go to the FCI. Robert had known that political influence played a major role, since 95 percent of the clinical associates at the FCI were from some eight schools, six of which were located on the east coast. Although he guessed that many capable interns and residents existed elsewhere, there was a clear prejudice for the coast's "pipeline" schools. This made his acceptance even more meaningful. He had made it completely on his own, against all odds.

For one of the rare times in his life, Robert had been afraid that he might not succeed. His interview with Dr. Free had gone well, but his interview with Dr. Frederick hadn't. He had been left with the disturbing sense that the latter might attempt to block his application to the FCI. Dr. Frederick had only grunted when Robert had talked about his rapport with cancer patients, and gave him the vague impression that Robert wasn't giving the answers that were expected. Maybe he should just have stuck to discussing his love for the lab - that is what he would be doing there, after all. But apparently Dr. Frederick had been sufficiently impressed with Robert's unusual answers. And so young Dr. Gordon, still in debt and getting used to the hectic life of the physician, was on his way to one of the most prestigious research institutions in the world.

"Read the letter to me, M M," he said with a shaky voice. And as she read the short note, images formed in his mind of the actual experiences that he would have at the FCI, the excitement of discovery, the joy of doing something to combat cancer, to someday help those stricken people who were ignored on so many hospital wards. His appointment was an opportunity not only to continue with his efforts to better understand the cancer problem at the bedside, but it would also allow him to develop the essential laboratory skills to pioneer new forms of cancer treatment.

Robert knew the field was moving very quickly. There were even rumors that President Nixon was going to launch a major federal effort against cancer, finally bringing this illness that struck a quarter of the population into the public eye. It reminded Robert of what had happened with kidney disease. Interest in these disorders had mounted dramatically following government funding for dialysis. Patients who previously were not "interesting teaching cases", as Dr. Xavier might say, because of terminal renal failure, suddenly became interesting to many professors, some of whom had changed their area of interest to nephrology when federal bucks had been channeled into research on kidney disease and renal dialysis. It was interesting what made a case "an interesting patient".

Robert suspected that a major government program in cancer funding would have the same impact, only on a much grander scale. An all-out "war on cancer" just might be coming. And he knew that his appointment to the FCI was critically important to his career.

He had made his commitment. And he was ready to meet the challenge.

CHAPTER 6

THE TASK FORCE

June 1980

It was cool, the sun an orange hue just beginning to light the Texas prairie. John always liked the last half mile of a run the best. He'd come winding around the large lilac bush, picking up speed because he knew it would soon be over, then finish a few yards from the huge circular drive that led up to the main house. He'd walk around the building, hands on hips and catching his breath, enjoying the spectacular landscaping and luxurious gardens at this, his favorite hour, when no one else was yet awake.

Usually John would go through the kitchen entrance and pour a glass of Perrier, then meander up the central stairway to his private bathroom in the west wing. He took a special pleasure in walking among the priceless antiques, plush carpets, and carefully placed dried flower arrangements when he was clad only in grubby Nike track shoes and wringing wet shorts. It made him feel like the only truly living thing in this palace of opulence. He'd climb the stairs, being careful not to touch the walls or even the banister, and then read the Wall Street Journal as he soaked in the jacuzzi the size of any normal person's bedroom for a half hour or so, until he began to hear some signs of life from elsewhere in the house.

But today was different. He could hear and smell the difference long before he could even see the kitchen entrance. When he entered, he saw starched white uniforms scurrying about, carrying platters and bowls and glassware. A huge black woman was barking directions in the middle of the chaos. He didn't recognize anyone. He thought for a wild moment that he had entered the wrong house. As he stood at the center of the commotion, ducking trays and trying in vain not to be noticed, one of the youngest of the white uniformed scurriers came up to him.

"Would you kindly get the hell out of here? Can't you see you're dripping all over the floor? Do you think I want to rewax it because of you?"

John's mouth fell open, but before he could answer, the boss lady grabbed her underling and whispered something to her. The young woman turned as red as a slice of bloody roast beef, and ducked out of the room. That was the last time she'd ever talk to John J. Owens.

With all eyes upon him, John made his way to the parlor, where his senses were literally assaulted by an ocean of flowers. The scent was so overpowering that he felt nauseated. More starched young women, and a few men, hovered over the flowers, lest a petal dare be out of place. Somewhere within the jungle that had once been his home he recognized the butler and an upstairs maid, and realized that he had indeed come into the right house.

It was still only 6:00 a.m., so he knew that his family would not be among the conscious for at least another hour, and his daughter Babsie, the object of all of this fuss, not until at least 10:00. So he thought he'd wander about and watch the ridiculous preparations for a bit before retiring to his bathroom.

What an incredible year it had been, his daughter's debutante year. Last June he had thrown her a huge high school graduation party, and tonight he was hosting a good, old-fashioned, downhome barbeque for his little girl, as only a wealthy Texan could. You'd think she'd at least be grateful, but not little Babsie. A barbeque was so common. Everyone had them. Why couldn't he have turned the ranch into a fiefdom, like Twinkles Cunningham's party, or Camelot, like Bambi Wellsworth's? The very least he could have done, if he really loved her, was to import a herd of zebra or build a riverboat. Something to make her stand out in the deb crowd. It was SO important!

John had asked her sarcastically if she would like him to have the Taj Mahal reconstructed over the bathhouse. As usual, she missed his point completely, and for a frightening moment, seemed to take him seriously. Quickly he told her that a barbeque at Five Aces ranch would just have to do. Although John could buy the Cunninghams and the Wellsworths over half a dozen times, he was quite fed up with the extravagances of being an oil family. Wasn't it enough that he had plunked down several thousand dollars for Babsie's ball gowns and designer dresses? It cost him more than $2000 a week to dress the kid! God forbid she should dare wear the same outfit twice in a year. Not to mention the team of social secretaries who were absolutely essential to arrange her dates for the year, to appropriately screen the young men, and to ensure that Babsie went to the right tea at the right time. He wondered if they told her when to go to the bathroom.

John loved his little girl dearly, but he hoped he would survive her debutante year. And once she came out, he didn't know quite where she was going. She was not exactly the stuff of which supreme court justices or Nobel-prizewinning scientists were made. He was well aware of all of the women's lib crap floating around during Babsie's teen years, but none of it had seemed to rub off on his daughter. All she wanted was to have a good time and eventually to meet a nice rich guy, and presumably make babies and spend money the rest of her life. He supposed that at age 18 that was all right, and after all, she'd never taken the opportunity to think much about what she might do with her life, because everything had always been done for her. But John had hoped that she'd develop an interest in something other than buying dresses and impressing Houston society with her monstrous wealth.

Why couldn't she be a little like his son? He had just finished his junior year at Rice, and was already thinking about graduate school. John was so proud of his boy, who since childhood had followed him around on the ranch and to the oil fields, always asking questions that increased dramatically in complexity as he grew older. Now he undoubtedly knew more about petroleum than I, John thought. It was no surprise when he had majored in geology, but the scope of his knowledge still amazed his father, who had been educated in the field. And no rich kid problems; his head was in the right place, ready to carry on for John J.

Realizing that there was nothing for him to do, John tiptoed up the stairs and went into his bathroom. The butler had already drawn his bath and placed the Journal and a selection of current magazines next to the toilet. John settled in on the throne - running always seemed to activate his intestines about a half hour after he stopped, and also sometimes during the run itself (that's what bushes were invented for). As John opened a Playboy magazine, he glanced downwards and noticed a slight brownish-red stain on his running shorts. Funny, that had happened a few weeks ago, too. He wondered if he should check it out. It was probably just his diet. He'd read in Runner's World that a heavy meat diet could cause blood in the stool, but what could he do about that in a place where breakfast was steak and eggs, lunch a bowl of chili, and dinner a pile of ribs? Nathan Pritikin would have no place in Houston, particularly on the Five Aces ranch.

John prided himself on his exemplary health. How many 53-year-olds could run a 10K in 39 minutes? He didn't smoke, and only drank on occasion, and made sure to get regular physicals. It was just three months ago that he'd passed his physical with flying colors. He wondered if he should bother telling Dr. Walstone about the blood, since he'd been so recently examined. Well, whatever he decided, he couldn't do anything about it until the absurd hullaballoo downstairs had blown over. He got into the jacuzzi and enjoyed what would probably be the last few peaceful moments of the day. The warmth enveloped him and his mind transcended time.

The great wealth of the Owens family dated back to a single night in 1900, September 9th. Three things of note happened on this date: one of the worst hurricanes in history tore through Galveston; a ranch hand named Owens won a worthless parcel of 125 acres in nearby Beaumont; and the ranch hand's wife gave birth to a 10-pound boy, William, as the eye of the hurricane passed overhead.

When William was a toddler, something else of import happened. A gusher that made all others look like trickles exploded from Spindletop field, in Beaumont. In a matter of hours, ranch man Owens, an intelligent but penniless man, became a wealthy oil baron.

Although educated only through the eighth grade, and that included more absences than presences, he had a sharp business sense that enabled him to oversee the extraction and refining of his oil, as he wisely invested profits into additional land. As his personal worth soared, he had the foresight to channel some of his earnings into other ventures, acquiring mineral mines, cattle, tankers, and timber.

And so young William, the first son to appear after three daughters, could not even remember a time when he did not have the best of everything at his fingertips. He had inherited his father's sense of practicality and realized that the Owens dynasty of tomorrow depended upon intelligent planning today. He too had forsaken formal training for an education in the fields, where, at his father's side, he learned every phase of every operation in which the family had invested. So involved was he in the makings and maintenance of the family fortune that he ignored the dozens of young lovelies who couldn't wait to sink their teeth into his bank account. By a miracle, he entered his twenties unhitched, and planned to stay that way for awhile.

But unfortunately William was not as careful a planner in his personal life as he was in the oil fields. In 1927, he got the young daughter of one of the gardeners pregnant. He simply could not resist her, especially that night when he had retired to his bedroom to find her lying in his bed, covered only with his quilt. They had been eyeing each other for weeks, and he knew that eventually they would get together. Get together they did, and the result was John J. Owens, born, like his pappy, under the eye of a hurricane in the summer of that year. A hushed-up civil ceremony shortly after a missed period ensured that the child was legitimate, and, more importantly, that he was the rightful heir to the Owens fortune.

Also unfortunately, the mother, spectacularly beautiful even towards the end of her pregnancy, died when John was born. All the wealth in the world could not stop her hemorrhaging. William was shocked but suffered no permanent damage from his wife's demise. John was quickly whisked away by a contingent of nannies and nurses, so he was completely unaware that he was without a mother.

On the day that John turned six months of age, he got a mother. William, under considerable paternal pressure (his mother, like most wise women of the day, knew when to keep quiet, which was most of the time), had married Louisa Prescott, the rather homely daughter of a successful cattle rancher who leased oil fields to the elder Owens. Louisa was pleasant, reasonably intelligent, and in short time had produced a daughter for William. She was a wonderful mother to both children, and she and William saw no need to tell John that she wasn't his natural mother. If William wasn't exactly head over heels in love with his wife, he did grow to cherish her and appreciate her goodness and competency in running a household. He grieved for months when she died of tuberculosis ten years after Olivia's birth.

John did little to become one of the richest and most powerful men in Texas. It was all done for him, thanks to a fortuitous poker game and the wits of his daddy and granddaddy. Nevertheless, he had inherited the family mental acuity, and eagerly joined the game of investing and expanding the fortune. He enjoyed the challenge of predicting which industries and endeavors might take off in the Houston area.

And the investments that turned out to be wise - such as backing that little bauxite mine in Karnes County - catapulted the family fortune even further.

By the 1950s, John had become a vital part of the Owens team which was still lead by a middle-aged William and his aged but still alert father. In the mornings John surveyed the family holdings, often driving to the gulf to check the refineries and transport activities. He spent his afternoons, particularly in the brutally hot summers, reading journals and reports in his never-ending search for new investments. And the evenings were spent at the deb parties and charity dinners and other bashes that made up the Houston social scene.

Although John wasn't a Harvard or Princeton man, the Owens name was so powerful that his lack of a formal education meant little. His tall lean body and boyish good looks meant a lot, at least to the debs. His wealth, of course, was what attracted their daddies. And so John J. Owens found himself a much-in-demand escort, and in those years he entertained so many proper and not-so-proper young ladies that he even mixed up their names at times.

But not Cassandra. He was struck speechless by her beauty the moment he met her. The youngest of four daughters, Cassie had been the skinny little kid who hid behind her sisters, so unnoticed that John did not even realize she existed until she seemed to materialize from nowhere at the age of 18, so stunning that the other debs faded in her presence. When he began to dance with her that first time, he was captivated when she spoke. She had a throaty voice that was simply intoxicating.

And to top it all off, Cassie was smart. She saw the whole debutante routine as a huge joke, and told John that she was just playing along to keep peace in her family. She read the newspaper every day, devoured books, and had somehow gotten far more out of her expensive European education than learning to play the piano and embroider. Best of all, she seemed just as enraptured with John as he was with her.

They married at the end of the deb season in 1954 in a storybook wedding that became a storybook honeymoon and marriage. After four years of ascending to the heights of Houston society, Cassie slowed down her hectic schedule of luncheons and charity events to get down to the serious business of baby-making. Their son arrived in 1958, and a daughter in 1960.

Meanwhile, John had seen to it that the family fortune continued to grow. He expanded into cotton, corn and rice, bought more mineral mines, and went into asphalt production. He purchased pulp and paper mills, started a highly mechanized chicken farm, and continued to add to his cattle holdings. He bought sheep and invested in a sweater company in New York. He dabbled in manufacturing, buying into a chemical plant near Dallas that produced nylon intermediates, methanol, and polyethylene resins for the textile and plastics industry. He owned five percent of the American Chemical Company, an innovative company in Connecticut. If it sounded the least bit interesting or promising, John J. Owens owned a part of it.

Yet another technological dabbling of John's began to bear fruit in the 1970s. A few years earlier he had invested in the Huxley Embryo Transport Company, largely because he liked the science-fictionish nature of what they were trying to do. The company's scientists had found a way to extract cattle embryos and implant them in rabbits, and then ship the rabbits to countries desiring the particular breed of cattle. It was far cheaper than shipping cattle, safer and easier than shipping sperm, and people were responding simply to the novelty of the idea. The company was also experimenting in freezing and shipping these embryos without "living incubators". John imagined a time when such embryo technology would be applied to humans - and, as usual, he would prove to be correct.

He was a very generous man. He paid his thousands of employees well, and not a few hospital wings, libraries and playgrounds bore his name. He contributed to a reforestation program, made endowments to all the Houston area colleges, and sent some of his house staff's children through school. John Owens became not only the richest man in Houston, but also one of the most-liked.

And so thanks to some initial luck, coupled with brains, foresight, and guts, by June 12, 1980, the date of the best barbeque the state of Texas would ever see (with or without the Taj Mahal), John J. Owens was twice over a billionaire.

John opened his eyes. He must have dozed in the bath. The Playboy centerfold was now floating in the tub. John dried himself off, got dressed, and headed down to the kitchen to see if he could grab something to eat from the mounds of delicacies that were piling up everywhere. Perhaps he'd even meet someone he knew.

He bumped into Cassie in the hallway. They had seen so little of each other lately, what with all of the social activities. Having a daughter was exhausting.

"Good morning, dear. Have you run already?" Cassie asked, glancing at her watch.

"Sure, it's nearly 8:00. You know I'd roast if I ran any later than 7:30."

"Well then, have you eaten?"

"Are you kidding? How?"

"I'm having some fruit and rolls sent to my sitting room. Why don't you join me. Let's stay away from this madness as long as possible," Cassie said, maintaining the sense of isn't-it-awful-but-don't-you-love-it-anyway that she had displayed at her debut so long ago.

John was only too happy to keep away from the crowd and to grab a few private moments with his wife. She was still so beautiful.

"So, Mr. Owens, how are you?" Cassie asked as she poured their coffee.

"Well, the uranium mine's picking up again, the ewes are producing well, oil prices are up, and the frozen embryo business is strong."

"I asked how YOU are."

"Oh. I don't know. I should be feeling all sentimental about Babsie's big day, but I just can't accept her attitude about the whole thing. What I do is never grand enough or original enough for her. She didn't even appreciate that the Charlie Daniels Band cancelled an important engagement to be here, as did the governor. What does she want - to transform the ranch into heaven itself?"

"Hey, that's not a bad idea!" Cassie joked. Then she became more serious. "I know what you mean. Barbara takes far too much for granted. And she can't see beyond the moment. I do so wish she'd give a little more thought to her future. It doesn't do nowadays for a woman to be totally dependent upon a man."

"Yes, I agree. Maybe after all this partying is over she'll mature a little."

"After the 'post-deb depression', I trust? Babs is already worrying about that, trying to line up the most popular psychiatrist for her inevitable breakdown."

"I've barely even seen her these last few weeks. What color is her hair?"

"Who knows?" shrugged Cassie, as they both laughed. "You won't even get to see her today. She wouldn't give up her daily routine for the barbeque tonight."

"What is this routine, I'm afraid to ask," said John.

"Well, the poor darling will be awakened at 10:00, and Missy will bring her breakfast in bed. Then, if she feels up to it, she'll write a few thank-you notes. Next, she'll dress, and then check over what has come back from the dry-cleaners, and perhaps see what's been sent over from Neiman-Marcus. Finally, she will check with her secretary on her dates."

"Oh dear, how does she cope with such responsibilities!"

"Let me continue, dear. Babsie will have luncheon, in her honor of course, at someone's home or the country club. I think it's the club today. Then she'll go shopping - after all, 3000 dresses are hardly enough for an 18-year-old. That will exhaust her, so she'll come home for a nap. She must rest up for the formal tea over at the Wellsworth ranch. Then maybe she'll phone some of her friends, to get the dope on who's wearing what tonight. And then she'll begin dressing for the barbeque. She's got a turn-of-the-century cowgirl outfit that's simply divine!" Cassie gushed sarcastically.

"My, she does lead a complicated life. I know it's all ridiculous, but it is fun spoiling her. I just hope we haven't ruined her completely in the process."

"Oh, I don't think so. She's still so young," Cassie said.

"Dear, there is a little something I wanted to mentioned to you," John started to say, but was interrupted by a loud knock at the door.

"Mrs. Owens, you must come downstairs immediately. The cakes have arrived and they're white - not blue like Missie Babsie requested," said a maid.

"Excuse me, dear. An emergency I suppose," said Cassie, as she gave her husband a quick kiss.

He had been about to tell her about the blood stain and ask her if she thought he should see Dr. Walstone. But there was no need to worry her. It was probably nothing.

The soiled running shorts turned out to be something!

The barbeque had gone off without a hitch, and dear Babsie had surprised herself by having a wonderful time. She had even thanked her daddy afterwards, an unusual gesture for someone who assumed that everything was simply due her. A day after the party, the house was once again spotless and relatively quiet.

John had eaten and drunk a little too much to consider going for a check-up the day after the barbeque, even though he had again found blood on his underwear. He became more concerned, even scared, and two days later he went to the doctor. He was asked to bring a morning stool sample, and, after a quick physical and a rectal exam, John was examined with a colonoscope, a flexible tube with a light that probed his rectum and colon, followed by a trip to the hospital for an unpleasant barium enema and x-rays of his colon. The procedures were painful and embarrassing, but worse than this was a sick fear that now gripped John's insides. He knew that blood in the stool could be a sign of cancer. He had never been ill in his life, and to be having his innards probed for something as devastating as cancer was unthinkable. This couldn't be happening to him. It just couldn't be!

But it was, and this afternoon John was to hear the results of the doctor's painful proddings.

This meeting began with some intense questioning by a nurse, something that did little to calm his nerves because she was quite attractive, and he didn't feel at all at ease discussing the details of his bathroom habits with her. But he recognized the seriousness of the matter and cooperated. No, he didn't know of any relatives who had colon cancer. Yes, there was some cancer, but he didn't think it was of the colon. Yes, he had been tired lately, but surely that was due to his daughter's extravagant social life and the preparations for her shindig. He was still recovering from it.

"What did you do about the fatigue?" asked the nurse.

"What any dedicated runner would do. I ran harder."

"Now that doesn't make any sense. Why didn't you cut back?"

"I'm in training for the Labor Day 10K. I didn't want to ease up. So it took me a few minutes more for a workout. Big deal. What does my fatigue have to do with anything?"

"You have been losing blood from your colon for several months. It has been enough to make you somewhat anemic. Not enough to send you to bed, but it could account for your loss of stamina."

"Oh. When can I see the doctor? I want to know what is going on!"

"The doctor will see you right away. Now please take a seat and relax, Mr. Owens."

"Sure."

"John, I'll be upfront with you. I don't like what the barium test showed."

"What? Be specific, Tom."

"Well, I can show you," the doctor replied as he put a dark x-ray sheet up on the light board. "The light colored tube is your large intestine, your colon. Notice how most of it is of the same width. But down here, on the right side, the diameter of the tube narrows considerably - see the darkened area? That's what we call a filling defect. The problem is on the right side. You haven't had any digestive symptoms, but there is definitely a blockage. Do you see it?" John shifted uneasily from one foot to the other, then cleared his throat. "Yes. What is the blockage, I'm afraid to ask?"

"That's what we have to get in there and see. The colonoscope showed that you have a few polyps, but they were not in the area of this large blockage, and they looked to me like the benign variety."

"So what's next?"

"I'd need to do another colonoscopy. I couldn't reach the right side this morning in the office because of the discomfort."

"But won't it hurt this time?"

"No, this time you'll be under light sedation. It's unpleasant, but bearable."

"How do you know? Have you had it done?"

"As a matter of fact, yes. The colonoscope will allow us to remove any small growths, plus view the entire large intestinal tract and take biopsies of any larger growths, particularly this area of blockage," he said as he pointed again to the obviously constricted right colon of John J. Owens, Texas billionaire.

"And what would happen if we didn't do this? Couldn't the growths just shrink on their own?"

"Some do that, but usually not those of the colon. Even if a growth is benign, it would enlarge until it blocks your intestine. And that would be a disaster."

"Oh. Can we do this soon? What happens if the big growth is, eh, a cancer?"

"We'd have to do a second procedure to remove it, and probably part of the intestine too."

"Would I have to wear one of those bag things?"

"Probably not. We can just reattach the cut ends of the intestine."

"By the way, who is 'we'?"

"As you know, I'm an internist. While I use a colonoscope and can make the diagnosis, the surgery, if it is necessary, requires a surgeon, a good one. And I have just the man in mind."

"The best. You know that cost isn't a problem."

"I'll schedule your colonoscopy at Houston Medical Center, and some other tests."

"Do I have to go in the hospital for them?" The sick feeling in his stomach rose to anticipate the answer.

"Yes, let's do it in the hospital to be sure the exam is complete."

July

John did some rapid shuffling of his schedule, making sure that his various farms, cattle operations, and oil rigs could function without him for a few days. Then, the next day he checked into Houston Medical Center.

He was right to expect the worst. The probing had seemed to take forever as he lay on his side in a dreamlike state. He was vaguely aware of the mutterings of the doctors who hovered over him, but didn't strain himself to hear their comments. John knew that a microscopic examination of the tissue was necessary to confirm cancer, which would take place while he was in his room, asleep. He stayed in the hospital overnight. In the morning, Dr. Walstone arrived to deliver the verdict. It wasn't good, but like most doctors, he started off with the "good" news.

"Good morning, John. How do you feel?"

"Fit as a fiddle and raring to go, as they say. But what do the pathologists say?"

"Well, we snared three small polyps which, as I had suspected, were dangling from stalks and were benign."

"And..." prompted the patient.

"And a fourth polyp didn't look so good. It was what we call a villous adenoma. It has sort of a fringe on it, and half of them are malignant."

"Spare me the medical lingo, but that sounds like bad news."

"The bad news comes from the biopsy of that large constriction we saw in your barium scan. I'm sad to say it contains malignant cells. We must go in to remove it at once."

"What does 'at once' mean?"

"Since you're here and the pre-op tests have been done, let's schedule you for tomorrow."

John was silent for a few seconds. He suddenly felt a wave of nausea. He was flushed with a pounding headache. He wanted to scream "GET THE HELL OUT OF HERE! GET OUT OF MY LIFE!" But he just muttered "Sure."

It had all happened so fast. A month ago he had been a healthy, active man of 53, enjoying his family, his businesses, his running. Today, he was in a hospital bed, keeping time by counting the frequency of post-surgery pain killing injections he received regularly. He forced smiles for his many visitors, and tried not to choke on the scent of the flowers that lined the room. They reminded him of a funeral home. He'd spent much of the time worrying whether the Owens empire would collapse without him, and he was growing quite annoyed at the nurses who continually pried the phone from him to check the IV or his privates.

They'd even sent in a social psychologist to allow him to open up his feelings about having cancer. How could he open up his feelings, whatever that meant, when it had hardly even sunk in that he had this illness? It was all impossible. They'd removed a few inches of his intestine, and that was that. The cancer was taken out, and all he had to do was to get his strength back. Right?

He'd been in the hospital a week now, and finally today they were taking out the nose tube and maybe even the IV. He would be a complete - well, almost complete - man again. His pain from the incision was minimal now, and he was itching to get back to work. Only three more days to go.

There was a knock on the door, and before he could utter a come-in, Dr. Walstone entered, followed by two nurses. They removed his nasogastric tube and the IV.

"Wow, I feel human again. So, how am I doing, Tom?"

"You tell me. How do you feel?"

"A little sore and a lot bored. Have you even watched one of these things?" he said as he pointed to the TV screen, where three actresses stood screaming at each other. "These stupid soaps are a form of anesthetic."

"I'm glad to see you've regained your sense of humor."

"Tom, no bull, how am I doing?"

"John, I've got some bad news. It was really quite unexpected, but it does happen."

"What are you talking about? Bad news about what? I thought this was all over," John asked haltingly.

"John, you asked earlier why the operation took four hours. And why we had to remove two feet of your colon if the tumor was only an inch in diameter. And why you had to have that bone scan."

"Yes ..."

"Well, the tissue surrounding the tumor suggested that the cancerous cells may have spread a little, so we removed more than we had expected to, plus the surrounding lymph nodes. Actually, it's a protective measure that's fairly routine."

"Go on." John propped himself up in the bed and nervously gripped the side railings.

"It's a good thing we removed as much as we did, because cancer cells were indeed found a few inches from the primary tumor."

"But if they were removed, there's no problem. Right?"

The doctor paused. And in the utter silence, John knew what had happened.

"Unfortunately, the cells have spread farther than the intestine. That extra hour you were on the table was spent searching your other abdominal organs. And we found a suspicious bit of tissue in your liver. We removed some of it," the doctor stated.

"You don't need to tell me the rest. Please leave."

This request was most unusual for the inquisitive and cooperative Owens, and Dr. Walstone was hesitant to leave at that moment. He started to object. But John waved him out, and the doctor could see that the powerful man, the richest man in Texas, had tears in his eyes.

"Okay, John. We'll talk another time. Please call me whenever you feel up to it. There is treatment."

And so John J. Owens, owner of a good-sized chunk of the second largest state in the Union, was left along with the funeral parlor flowers, the Wall Street Journal and a pile of Business Weeks, and the incessant chattering of the soap opera bimbos.

He snapped off the TV, swept the clutter from his bed, pushed away his phone, and began to utter deep, heaving sobs.

John's grieving lasted the remainder of his hospital stay. Dr. Walstone filled Cassie in on the details of his illness, and what needed to be done in the future. John did not want to discuss his condition at all, and as a result, Cassie knew much more about what would happen to him than he did. But that was the way he wanted it, at least for now. It was unreal, like a dream. He just wanted to go home.

Once back at the ranch, John buried himself in his bedroom with financial reports and a telephone. Within a few days he felt remarkably better, and was able to conduct his business over the phone. A week after his homecoming he could walk about a mile, and he looked forward to increasing that amount gradually each day. Cassie walked with him, and they talked about news events and the lives of their children and the latest scandalous stories in the Houston social scene and the space shuttle program. They talked about everything except John's cancer.

Cassie was worried about his refusal to face up to the situation, and had tried to get him to talk to her, had even suggested a psychiatrist to help him deal with this. John had balked - it was his liver that was out of kilter, not his head! She had more or less expected that response, and was actually relieved to see that her husband hadn't quit. So she decided to plunge right in herself.

She picked a beautiful sunny afternoon when Babsie was out at her zillionth tea (nothing had changed for her) and their son was in Galveston visiting one of the Owens' computer facilities. Most of the servants were napping - about the only logical thing to do when the mercury hit 96 ddegrees. Cassie pulled up a chair next to John's recliner in his air-conditioned bedroom, and dove right in.

"John, we have to talk."

"Don't tell me. You are having affairs with twelve men and want your freedom."

"John, please be serious. We have so much to discuss."

"I don't want to talk about death."

"Neither do I. I want to talk about life. Your life. And mine."

"What do you mean? You know damn well that cancer that has metastasized to the liver is a slow death sentence. How do you like that? I've even learned the correct words," he said bitterly.

"It doesn't have to be. There are new treatments coming out every day. Every patient can be treated, even you. Especially you. You can't give up, because that's giving in to it."

"What are you saying? Is there a treatment? Did Tom say something?" John began to look more animated.

"Well, for now they want to start you on some chemotherapy. And there are other options."

"Go on ..."

"You're a powerful man. Think about it. Three hospitals in this state have wings named after you, and another two have your libraries. Remember those biomedical training grants you established? The endowments? I've been checking into our holdings, and you've funnelled several million dollars into the biomedical field right here in Houston, not to mention your contributions elsewhere."

"I'm beginning to get your idea," said John as he shifted about on the recliner.

"I have a suggestion. While you're convalescing - and midsummer is a horrible time to be out anyway - why don't you do a thorough evaluation of the entire Owens enterprise, and see just what it is you are supporting. Who knows, you might already be funding some hot young researcher who is on the verge of curing colon cancer."

"That's right!" John said excitedly.

"And if you're not already funding such a project, you can start one. Or many. Who needs another computer company, and to hell with the aerospace industry. Why, we can fund someone to work with your own cancer, to find the answer to your disease."

John was already out of the chair, pacing the room, looking almost like his old self. Cassie could see that his mind was already racing way past hers.

"Cassie, my darling Cassie. You've just given me back the chance of my life." She fell into his arms and he held her to him tightly. "Now, go and get me that listing from the Howard A. Miller Foundation that came in the mail last week. It's still on my desk."

A few minutes later Cassie returned with a tray of cool drinks and the listing. John grabbed it from her and leafed through the pages listing the research projects funded by the multimillion dollar foundation.

"What language is this in, anyway? What the hell are ketenethioacetals, or mitochondrial RNAs or glycosphingolipids? And what on earth is a smectide clay? That sounds positively obscene. I can't even tell if the research has to do with anything living or not. Cassie, would you go down and get a biology text from the library?

The were both so excited that they forgot that they had servants to do their errands. Cassie practically slid down the banister to the section of the library reserved for basic texts on all of the sciences and fledgling technological fields. This was the most life she had seen in John since the whole dreadful cancer problem -- she'd do anything to keep it going. Quickly, she pulled the tome from the shelf and ran upstairs with it.

"Thank you. Now, I'll read some things aloud and you look up what I don't understand. Let's see. 'Fungal asexual reproduction' -- that certainly biological, but not of much use to a human with cancer. Here's 'the biochemistry of pigments in the dinoflagellates' -- studying the color of dinosaurs won't help me a bit. Cass, look up 'transferrin'." He paused as he scanned the pages.

"Transferrin. It's a protein found in the liver."

"Great! I'll just star this project and I'll get in touch with them. I hope it isn't rat livers though. Moving along... 'Comparison of the DNA sequence of the actin gene family in the sea urchin, macaque and human.' Do you think that would have anything to do with cancer? Here's something that sounds exciting: 'Cell aggregation patterns in Dictyostelium discoideum.' Cell aggregation. That could have something to do with the behavior of cancer cells, don't you think? Look up this dicty business."

"Okay." A pause as she shuffled through the gigantic book, then frowned. "I don't think you want to hear this."

"Go ahead, what does it mean."

"Dictyostelium discoideum is a cellular slime mold. See, here's a picture." She handed him the book.

"What!" John exploded, throwing the book down. "You mean I'm sitting here with cancer cells invading my body and some jerk is playing around with a smear of snot growing under a log -- for a million bucks! What the hell is going on in biomedical research anyway? Whatever happened to doing things for people, with people? Who gives a good goddamn for fungus and dinosaurs and macaques and slime molds. What the..."

"Dear, don't you think we're going about this in the wrong way? You may be the wealthiest man in Texas, but you're not qualified to judge the quality of these projects, nor which might relate to cancer. Why don't you hire someone to help us?"

John was silent for a moment. He closed the Miller Foundation book.

"That's not a bad idea. And not a person. A committee. A task force. The John J. Owens Cancer Research Task Force. Who should we get? Lots of doctors, maybe a scientist or two?"

"Why don't you start with someone who can sift through all of the information on the research activities at M.D. Anderson and in the Texas university system?"

"That's a great idea, but why limit it to Texas? I'll scour the whole world if I have to. Certainly someone, somewhere is looking at colon cancer. Why can't they look at mine?"

Life seemed to have returned to John. He couldn't sleep. This idea, then that, rocketed through his head. He thought of all the people he knew who might help. Who he could hire. A strategy was forming in his overactive mind.

The next day, he assigned two of his vice presidents of Owens Oil to stop what they were doing and set up a Task Force, Think Tank, whatever the hell they wanted to be called. "Get me one of those onco-guys from M.D. Anderson, a cell biologist, and send over a rep from Owens computers, the R&D branch over near Beaumont. Send someone who knows how to do computer searches. I'll call Carlton Stinson, the head man at M.D. Anderson, myself."

The day after that, the Task Force met for the first time. John explained that their short-term goal would be to identify existing research projects dealing with colon cancer in people, and then make some contributions. Each member had been told beforehand of John Owens' health problem, and hence the impetus for the Task Force. The long-term goal, which John had not mentioned to anyone besides his wife, would be to persuade these researchers to use his own cancer cells in their work. And if nobody was interested, he would have to generate the interest. A few hospital wings or grants in the right places should do the trick. By God, he would make it happen.

On the advice of Chet Carpenter, the oncologist assisting the Task Force (whom John had met and been impressed with following his surgery), the computer jockeys started their search of the Federal Institutes of Health, including the FCI, the National Science Foundation and Howard A. Miller Foundation grants with the three letters "oma" in the title of the project. They began in Texas. And while the search indeed turned up a few relevant carcinomas, it also led to melanomas, gliomas, and other cancers that did not directly apply to John's case. It also turned up the word "hybridoma" several times, and Dr. Carpenter had mysteriously asked them to highlight these studies. The doctor suggested they focus the computer search on "carcinoma." Doing a dual search for 'carcinoma' and 'colon' or 'metastasis' and 'liver' might also help, he'd suggested. And after a few days, 49 promising Texas projects were identified.

Meanwhile, John stopped his letter writing and phone calling only to sleep and eat. He contacted Dan Weil over at American Chemical in Connecticut -- he hadn't pumped all of that money into their pharmaceutical ventures for nothing. He learned the bad news that Daniel was fighting a similar problem, lung cancer. He badgered Massachusetts General because a cousin of a friend had had a colon cancer treated there. He appealed to every politician he could find. He called anyone he heard of who was every remotely associated with the FCI. He clearly needed help in his search. There had to be a cure out there and he had the resources to find it.

So the Task Force added a few graduate students from the M.D. Anderson Tumor Cell Biology program to help in tracking down important studies -- they had the knowledge, would receive credit for their work, and were accustomed to very long hours. Each of the four grad students was given a short list of projects and was sent to the phone and the library. And what they found was not very encouraging. The 'surface antigen instability in carcinoma of the colon cells' that had intrigued Dr. Carpenter turned out to be in guinea pigs. And the 'metastatic patterns of colon cancer' that had attracted his attention was valuable only if you happen to be a mouse. The list went on. In the end, only 7 of the 49 identified cancer research programs were working with human material.

"What the hell is going on here?" Owens had bellowed when the students had reported to him. "Doesn't anybody care about people anymore?"

"Sir, it is both standard and necessary to work on animal models before attempting experimental procedures on humans," said one of the students.

"But people need help NOW. Who gives a flying fuck about goddamn monkeys and mice? Wait till the press gets ahold of this," John shouted to no one in particular, although the contingent of students, particularly the bold young man, were trying to quietly fade into the wallpaper. "Carpenter, I want you to visit each of the Texas researchers we've identified. Find out who is in charge of each project, we don't want to waste any time talking to anyone but the best. Start packing -- some are local and some not. You'll need to make two stops at the UT Health Science Center in Dallas, one here at M.D. Anderson and one at Rice, then UT Austin, Southern Methodist, and Texas Christian. I don't care what order you do them in -- just get on it now." He paused to put all the papers together. "Thank you, all of you. And I apologize for my outburst. You can leave now," he said as he mentioned to the students "but Carpenter, you stay."

There was a moment of silence as the members of the John J. Owens Cancer Research Task Force filed out of the room. "Chet, we need to expand. I need you full time now. Put on another physician or some Ph.D.s, whatever you think is best. Never mind the cost. Round up some more of those grad students -- pay off their Ph.D. programs to let them work for me full time. Those kids have fresh perspectives on things. Also, get some more computer whizzes. With all of this animal bullshit, we need to do searches for human metastatic carcinoma of the colon in the whole country, No, make that the world."

August

Chet Carpenter accepted. With his Task Force spreading its wings throughout the world cancer research community, John was now completely recovered from his surgery and was running three miles a day. He was fully back to the business of Owens Enterprises. He began to spend more and more time reading up on cancer and the different types of treatments available. He knew about the traditional surgery and chemotherapy with 5-fluorouracil. He had read about radiation. But he also looked into the unconventional treatments -- laetrile, the Symington method of positive mental imaging, macrobiotic diets, literally everything that was out there, including coffee enemas, megavitamins and lentil beans, and the secret serums. A real witch's brew. He grew nervous waiting for Carpenter to check in.

Dr. Carpenter returned from his Texas tour on August 12, and he and John met in his plush underground offices at the Five Aces. John appeared to be in the prime of health, but the strain that he was under was evident in his eyes.

"Well, don't keep me guessing. What happened? Start with the most promising; I'm not in the mood for disappointment."

"I'm sorry to depress you, but I really don't have much to report," the doctor began.

"What do you mean? Aren't those guys doing what they're paid to do?"

"Yes, they are, but not very much during the month of August. That's the only month professors don't have students underfoot, and most of them like to get away to conferences or vacations."

"Didn't you speak to anyone? How can scientific research just shut down? My cancer isn't stopping just because it's August. Don't they deal with living, breathing, human beings? PEOPLE!"

"Oh, the labs don't shut down. But most of the principals were out. Mainly, I talked to post-docs."

"What the hell is a PI? And a post-doc?"

"A PI is a principal investigator -- you've funded a bunch of them. That's what happens to the money you donate to research. And a post-doc is short for 'post-doctoral research associate' -- someone who's between being a student and a big-shot. They are often the source of ideas and breakthroughs, and they do the work," Carpenter explained.

"Oh," Owens responded a bit sheepishly. "Well, what did the post-docs have to say?"

"When they heard I was an oncologist interested in tumor cell biology of metastatic colon cancer they were interested, and described their research. And when I mentioned that the Foundation I represented might have some funds available if the research would take a particular avenue, they grew more interested. But when I told them which way we wanted the research to go -- to use your cells to try to search for a specific solution for you -- they all backed away."

"What do you mean?"

"Some of them became defensive, even insulted. As if I was trying to buy them out. Made comments about research for the benefit of all, and using standard cell lines and such."

"They do work with human material, don't they?" John asked. "Well, where do they get it?"

"You can get human cell cultures from a number of places. It's a rather standard procedure."

"Like where? What do they do, rob graves? Wait around for some poor soul to donate his body to science?"

"Well, one place, believe it or not, is the Human Cell Bank in Medwell, New Jersey."

"You've got to be kidding. That sounds like something out of the twilight zone."

"Possibly, but it's very much a part of the real world. You can even order cells out of a color-coded catalog, and charge it to your grant number. We use them over at Anderson."

"So what are you waiting for?"

"What do you mean?"

"Get my cells in there!" John jumped up in his excitement.

"It's not that easy."

"Now what do you mean?"

"We have to get the cells. That'll mean a liver biopsy. Another hospital stay."

"If I have to, I have to. Get the cells, then present this thing as if we're doing the cell bank a big favor -- send them a donation, while you're at it. Then go back to those labs and convince the PIs to use my cells. It's simple."

"John, you have to understand. Most researchers work on the general problem of cancer as if cancers are all alike. They don't research an individual's cancer to try to develop treatment for that patient. And John, there's one more thing."

"Yes?" John asked distractedly.

"Everyone I spoke with, after I mentioned your personal plight, suggested you contact the FCI."

"What can they do? I've heard that you die of your cancer while you're waiting for them to evaluate you."

"But you're not just Joe Schmoe. Don't you have any connections there?"

"Of course I do. I've already tried that. They were very nice, but not very encouraging. But I'll try again. Maybe I'll get someone who will really listen to me, or who appreciates the value of money. Thanks a lot, Chet."

John's curiosity was piqued by the mention of the FCI, and just for fun he thought he'd try getting through to them as Joe Schmoe. After Carpenter left his office, John dialed 1-800-4-CANCER, the hotline number written on several of the pamphlets he had been reading.

"Federal Cancer Information Hotline, may I help you?" asked the clear, feminine voice.

"Yes, I have colon cancer and would like some information."

"Hold on one moment, sir. Someone will be right with you." Click. Several minutes of Muzak.

"Hello, can I help you?" chirped a voice nearly identical to the first.

"Yes, I have colon cancer and I'm interested in participating in a clinical trial."

"Please hold again, sir." Click. Muzak. A longer wait this time. John grew impatient.

"Yes, may I help you?" another similar voice said.

"You must be triplets," John growled. "Yes, you can help me. I have colon cancer," he almost shouted, prepared to slam down the receiver if he was put on hold again.

"Where are you calling from, sir?"

"Why do you need to know?"

"The FCI sponsors trials here in Washington, but also at centers throughout the country. We also have a number of trials involving colon cancer. Maybe you live near one of our centers."

"I live in Houston."

"That's good. We have a few trials at some of the university medical centers there. Let me send you a packet on our programs. Can I have your name and address?"

"No, not just yet." John didn't know why he was uneasy about obtaining this information. Perhaps he was just not used to doing things the way ordinary people did, without special treatment. And he found it hard to admit to a strange voice on a phone that he had cancer. He could always call back. "Could you just give me some information now?"

"Certainly. What would you like to know?"

"How does someone get into one of your programs?"

"You have to have a type of cancer that is being studied in a particular project, and be in good health otherwise."

"Oh. But what if I have a type of tumor that is not being studied?"

"Then you will be put on a list and matched up to an appropriate program when one arises."

"And what if more people apply for a program that can be accommodated? How do you choose?"

"Well, the researchers have some say in who gets chosen. But basically, its a first-come-first-serve situation, provided you meet the selected criteria."

"You mean I could get wait-listed, like waiting on an airplane seat?"

"Yes, it's the only fair way."

"That's easy for you to say. You mean to tell me that a famous person, or one with a lot of money to donate to cancer research, couldn't get in ahead of a nobody from Peoria? What about a senator? Or a ballplayer or movie star?"

"Our policy is first-come-first-serve, no favors. Would you like me to send you some information on selection of patients for clinical trials?"

"No, that won't be necessary just yet. But could I talk to an FCI researcher about my cancer, now?"

"I'm afraid that's impossible. We are fully trained nurses who can handle any questions about FCI policy over the phone."

"Well, thank you for your time."

Clearly, this wasn't the way to go. What happened to those poor slobs with cancer who didn't have any money or know anybody? He'd make a large donation to the FIH and earmark if for the FCI, then maybe he'd get past the 800 number and their specially trained nurses. But maybe money wasn't the answer. Maybe they'd listed more to political influence. He'd call Sebastian March, the distinguished Senior Senator from Texas. And Senator Daniels, he had helped him get re-elected in a tight race a decade ago. Owens support had taken them to Washington. They damn well owed him!

September

By the time that the annual heat spell began to dissipate over the Texas range, John was feeling quite well-- even running about five miles a day. But things were not going well in his effort to find himself a cure. After calling the FCI as Joe Schmoe, John had made a $500,000 donation to the FIH patient fund, then requested a meeting with officials at the agency. He had been given a royal treatment by the slick PR people, even a tour of some of the research and clinical facilities, but hadn't located a clinical trial that looked promising for him. Well, at least they knew that he, and his cancer, existed.

He did the same at the Sloan-Kettering Memorial Cancer Center in New York City, and flew up to Roswell Park in Buffalo shortly thereafter, and then to the Dana Farber Cancer Institute associated with Harvard. At each institution, he made generous donations and not-so-subtle requests that research into his particular type of cancer be stepped up. He even "offered" to donate his own cells for the research effort.

But there were no takers. All he heard was FCI trial over and over again, until he felt like he was going in circles.

He'd also tried the Houston office of the American Cancer Society, where the office crew had been thrilled by his visit and did their damnedest to extract as much money from him for their cause -- never suspecting that it was his personal cause, as well. By this time he had read a great deal, and quickly realized that the ACS staff, although dedicated and successful fundraisers, knew little, if anything, about what they were raising bucks for. Hell, the woman in charge didn't even know what metastasis meant when he had mentioned it. Let them stick to their charity events. The answer would come from a laboratory, not from a bunch of chattering, if well-meaning volunteers.

October

In early October, tragedy struck the Owens family. John's sister, Olivia, was killed in a car accident. Her head had smashed into the windshield at 60 miles per hour. She died instantly, according to her husband. But, the body continued to live with artificial support, waiting for a medical death pronouncement and the possibility of organ donation.

Olivia and her husband lived with their two children in Virginia where she had taught high school and he was a dentist. Even though she and John saw each other infrequently, they wrote and spoke often on the phone, maintaining the close ties of childhood.

John was by this time so obsessed with conquering his illness that even while he mourned his beloved sister, he thought of a way that she might be able to help him, even in death. He called his father and brought him downstairs. Yes, he knew it was late, but this could be a matter of life and death. The old man probably was too upset to be asleep anyway.

"A transplant? Do they do those sorts of things for cancer?" William had asked.

"I don't know, but why not? The cancer's been removed from my gut, but spread to my liver. Why not just replace the damn thing? And who could be a better donor than my sister -- may she rest in peace. Isn't it best when organ donors and recipients are closely related?"

"I don't think that would be a very good idea," his father answered, obviously disturbed.

"Why not? Is it that you don't want to disturb Olivia's body? She would be happy if somehow her senseless death could prevent someone else's, especially her own brother's."

"That's the whole problem."

"What is? Disturbing her body?"

"No. John, I hope you won't be angry for our never having told you this, but you and Olivia are only half brother and sister."

John was silent as the information sunk in. No. It couldn't be. His beloved mother in an affair and passing Olivia -- or God forbid, himself -- off as William's? No. That couldn't happen in his family. Maybe she was raped, and then couldn't bring herself to have an abortion. But then who was his father? He was suddenly confused, and didn't know what to say.

"Let me explain before you imagine all sorts of things." his father prompted. And then he told John of his natural mother, who had died giving birth to him. We saw no need to burden you with the knowledge of how your natural mother died. After all, you were still an infant when we were married. Please John, please understand."

John remained silent, absolutely shocked, yet relieved that there had been no wrongdoing, only actions to protect him. Tears in his eyes, for Olivia, for his parents and their secret, and for his own uncertain future, father and son embraced in their grief and fear. Of course, a transplant was out of the question.

November

By late fall, John Owens decided to take matters more into his own hands. The Task Force continued to track down promising research projects and to use the Owens fortune to being new ones. But while they were doing this, John himself took to springing surprise visits on some of the labs doing cancer research. The professors learned to recognize his bounding step in the hallways and to make themselves scarce at his approach. All lab personnel were told just what they could, and couldn't tell the generous but overbearing Mr. Owens. And so the increasingly desperate man was faced with a highly effective communications blockade.

Maybe he was mistaken in aiming at the top, at the guys who ran the labs and solicited donations. Maybe the trick was to grab the young talent. Were they hungry, more easily persuaded with money? And weren't the grad students and post-docs the scientists of tomorrow? Why not tap their brains today?

John hired a public relations and research team to look into the talent of tomorrow. The team scanned scores on the Graduate Record Exam which college seniors take for entry into Ph.D. programs in the biomedical sciences. All those who scored above the 95th percentile in biology and had applied to graduate programs related to cancer were sent a personal letter from John J. Owens, detailing a $40,000 predoctoral grant that he would provide, if the student did his or her thesis work on metastatic carcinoma of the colon, with the stipulation that Owens' cells be used. And even though a few interested students contacted him, the institutions to which they applied did not think that such directed research so early in a young scientist's career was for the student's benefit.

The team had a little more success in a similar granting program aimed at recent Ph.D.s whose theses passed the Task Force's now finely-honed computerized "oma" test. There were a few takers here, but they were still writing their grant proposals to Owens and attempting to find institutions that would allow them to carry out their research. It would be months before any actual work on his cancer could begin. He might not have months.

1981

In March, John's frenetic and increasingly desperate pace had to slow, as he became more tired than he had ever felt in his life. He thought at first that it was due to his crazy schedule, all the flying and arguments. He still couldn't fully accept that he was not healthy, despite the intensity of his actions to buy a cure. But when his breathing became labored after he had run only a half mile, aand his fatigue grew worse, he checked back into the M.D. Anderson Tumor Institute (he hated the stupid name -- it made him imagine a group of disgusting lumps sitting around in beds).

The news wasn't good. A new growth in what was left of his colon had ulcerated, leading to blood loss that had caused his anemia and lethargy. And worse, cancer cells were found in fluid pockets that had formed around his lungs and on his lower spine. He was given radiation treatments and started on a course of chemotherapy, and the new growth in his colon was scraped out.

The day after his surgery, John was visited by Patricia Babcock, a recently appointed member of the Task Force who was working on a doctorate in social psychology. Her credentials John thought, easily qualified her to evaluate the sometimes bizarre cancer treatments that people came up with. He also enjoyed her offbeat sense of humor, and he was much cheered when he saw her pretty blond head peek into his room.

"Come on in Pat. I'm bored to tears. Tell me something interesting."

"I've got quite a list for you this time, boss. Shall I read it aloud, or would you like to take a look?"

"I'm still capable of reading. Let me see it," he said with a smile as he reached for the pad of paper in her hand and studied it. "What the hell is this? Elephantopus elatus? What do happy elephants have to do with cancer?"

"Let me explain..." Patricia began, but John wouldn't give her a chance.

"And what the blazes is Catharanthus roseus? A social disease?"

"That's a Madagascar periwinkle sir," Patricia answered quietly. "And the first is a plant too."

"Pat, I don't need a salad or bouquet. I need something to stop my cancer. What is all of this bullshit anyway? It looks like those ridiculous studies on dinosaurs and sea urchins and slime I found when we started this whole thing."

"If you'd let me explain. The plants on my list, and the chemicals in them that I've highlighted, are Chinese medicinals that indeed destroy cancer cells."

"And how do they do that?"

"Most of them do it by preventing rapidly dividing cells from dividing. That zaps cancer cells, but it also affects healthy cells that normally divide rapidly, such as bone marrow cells and those that line the digestive tract, even hair cells. That's why chemotherapy often has side effects."

"Go on."

"Mr. Owens, many powerful drugs are synthesized by chemists only after they have studied the compounds which Mother Nature has already put into plants. Some potent anti-cancer drugs have been developed this way."

"Such as?"

"Have you heard of vincristine? Yes? It's derived from the Madagascar periwinkle."

"Well, I'll be. You certainly have done your homework. I do apologize! But how do you expect me to take you seriously after that report two weeks ago?"

"Which one was that?"

"You know, about the Greek researchers injecting dessicated sheep placenta, and the French quacks who grind up aborted human embryos?"

"People are really doing that, sir. And I did advise you that Dr. Carpenter said to stay away from that sort of thing."

"What about the eye of newt and frog leg potion cooked up in Tralfamador?"

"Okay, I did make that one up. I was trying to cheer you up a little. I'll try to be more serious -- that is, I know that this is a very serious endeavor. And I do hope that you are feeling better soon."

"Thank you. That'll be all for now. I appreciate your coming to see me. Good luck in tracking down some more cure-alls."

Two days later, Cassie took John back to the Five Aces. She hoped that the pleasant smells of spring would lift his spirits. Remembering how she had taken his mind off of his troubles a year earlier, she had already piked his bed high with portfolios of many of the emerging biotechnology companies. She knew they were just the thing to keep John's hopes up, his mind whirling. The exciting ideas coming from companies with such colorful names as Genentech, Biogen, and Cetus would certainly bring him back.

And once again, Cassie was right. Maybe these new companies were the answer, John thought aloud as he perused the folders. They were run by young people, and the reports mentioned substances that sounded different from the standard cancer drug names he had grown used to, all those "ycins." One in particular stood out -- interferon. With a name like that, whatever it was, it had to do something. He'd have to have someone check it all out. In the meantime, he'd buy as much stock as he could, right away, and start writing some letters. There wasn't any time to be lost now.

Two hours later, he put down his pen in exhaustion. He had drawn up a list of companies, contacts and ideas. Tomorrow he'd start in on the phone, or perhaps have someone from the Task Force do it. This time, he thought, he was really on to something. And once again, Cassie had saved the day, just as she had a year ago.

Could all of this have been going on a full year already? And what had he accomplished? Given away millions, and here he lay, his disease spreading, and he was helpless to stop it. Could he indeed do anything, or was he just squandering whatever time was left him?

As John began to drift into sleep, he was startled by the phone. Anxious for some contact with the outside world, he picked it up before the staff could do so.

"Hello, May I speak with Mr. Owens?"

"This is he. Who is calling?"

"Hello Mr. Owens. My name is Dr. Lizzard. I am the director of cancer therapy at the FCI."

John immediately sat up in bed and grabbed the pad and pencil on the table. He listened intently for several minutes jotting a few things down. "Yes, Dr. Lizzard. I understand. A new drug, new program. Yes, of course I'm interested."

John listened for several more minutes, while he frantically pushed on the buzzer near his bed to summon Cassie. She flew into the room, and stood by expectantly while he finished the conversation.

"Yes, yes. I'll be there tomorrow. Thank you so much."

And then John J. Owens, the most powerful man in Texas, hung up the phone, embraced his wife, and cried like a baby.

CHAPTER 7

NOBEL AMBITIONS

August 1979

George Trumpey was worried.

The short, balding Australian seemed almost lost behind the mountain of clutter on his desk, studying the draft of the paper he planned to send to the Journal of Science (JS). He knew that months and months of tedious research had gone into the seven pages, and that the work was quite important, but he felt just the slightest hesitation about publishing it. Was it premature? But the work going on elsewhere at the FCI gave him little choice. Hell, he had no time to wait. In this incredibly competitive field of virology, it wasn't so much the depth of one's work that was important, but whether or not it was the first to be published. And if Trumpey was to stick to his plan to become the best known virologist at the FCI, he couldn't let Roger Salla and his damn human lymphoma virus stand in the way.

He didn't really like throwing his weight around at JS, but nonetheless, he picked up the phone. The holy peer review system went straight to hell when competing labs had something to report. Trumpey knew that an FCI paper would certainly bump less important reports -- which was most everything. "Forced Copulation of Mallards in an Urban Population" would just have to wait another week to stun the world in this most coveted journal for scientists. But bumping ducks wasn't enough. If he put in a special word now, talked directly to the editor, his paper would appear in a scant four weeks. He supposed he wouldn't like the system very much if his life work was devoted to the mating rituals of ducks and he had finally gotten the beasts to do enough to publish, but this was cancer research. It had to come first. And anyway, they did this sort of thing over at JS all the time.

Trumpey hung up the phone before dialing, though, because he heard a commotion out in the reception area. But before he could extricate himself from the piles of paper threatening to cascade all over his robust middle, the bellowing grew closer and the door burst open to reveal a red faced, enraged Roger Salla, screaming so loud that Trumpey feared he would have a heart attack right there in his office. Salla was tall and angular, and on the rare occasions when he showed his feelings, looked a little like Frankenstein. And he had a reputation for barging into offices.

Today he wasted no time. "George, you ugly fat son of a bitch. I've got the goods on you now, and I'm gonna expose you to the world. Better watch the 6:00 news for this one!"

Trumpey treated the Frankenstein monster as he did his children -- he touched Salla's arm and spoke slowly and quietly. "Roger, close the door. You are making a scene. Everybody is listening."

Roger ripped away his colleague's hand and slammed the door. "George, I know and you know you've tried to ruin me in the past. I know and you know that one of your technicians has tried to spike my cultures. And I know and you know you have used every possible trick to discredit me. But now, by God, I've got you!" He paused to catch his breath and it looked to George as if the collective frustration of all their years of competition was finally boiling out. His face was bloated, the blood vessel across his right temple looked as though it might burst, and his eyes were bloodshot.

George suspected that Roger, known for his paranoia and penchant for James Bond movies, thought that one of his technicians was a spy. Salla ran his lab like a field marshal commanding an army and any hint of irregularity drove him crazy. Although George had no part in this particular bit of intrigue, he was amused, and decided to listen and egg his colleague on a bit.

"I've just squeezed the truth out of Sally Ryan. I caught her in the lab at night mixing bacteria into my tissue culture flasks!

I scared her into admitting that this wasn't the first time she'd done that -- she's been up to it for three years! And you and I both know what happened three years ago."

"Surely you're not suggesting..."

"You're damn right I am. It's perfectly obvious now how that jerk Sally can afford such ritzy clothing on a technician's salary!"

"Roger, settle down," George said, offering a seat. "You know there's not a thing you can prove. Sally has a long history of being into this difficulty and that, and you took a known risk in hiring her. She doesn't work for me or anyone else, she's just a crazy female -- and you're crazy for thinking there are spies lurking behind every incubator! Old Sally is just a frustrated technician who wanted to be a Ph.D. So she takes out frustrations on someone -- you -- who has what she wanted. It's really very common. Chances are she would spike cultures, if the price was right. More likely she would do it because you pissed her off over some issue. But as to her being my agent -- that is ridiculous!"

But George was alarmed just a little. Although Sally wasn't his plant -- she was too stupid and erratic for him to even consider using her -- the situation was startingly similar to what had happened three years earlier with the human leukemia virus. And then he had been involved. He'd arranged for someone to contaminate Salla's precious human leukemia cell cultures with gibbon virus. The result was a famous story at the Institute.

After a great deal of work and secrecy, Roger Salla had announced to the world that he had discovered the long-sought leukemia virus (HLV). To much fanfare, the discovery was hailed as preliminary, but possibly one of the great moments in the Federal Cancer Program. Roger played out his hero fantasy for six weeks, and then his star crashed. In trying to confirm Salla's result, a collaborator typed and retyped the virus. It wasn't from a human at all, nor did it cause leukemia.

It was standard laboratory virus from a gibbon, an ape!

Roger had suffered a considerable loss of prestige, and George actually felt a little badly, for the man was an aggressive and brilliant researcher, but his own work was more important. He couldn't let someone else, no matter how talented, finish first. Fortunately, most of the scientific community assumed that Salla was so excited by the results that he simply hadn't done enough in the way of verification studies before the announcement. What with all the FCI internal pressure to look good to the public and Congress, this was not surprising. Only George knew the true story, and of course, the technician who actually did the deed and had moved on. So Roger's saga of Sally the sloppy spy was all too familiar.

Roger wasn't finished. "I'm going to have your fat ass dragged before Musso by your stinking lab coat. Remember this day, George, for it marks the end of your scientific career!" he shouted, his face still an unhealthy looking red.

George again assumed the condescending tone he took with the boys. "Roger, sit down and be quiet. Haven't you damaged your scientific reputation enough without adding hysteria and paranoia to it? You can't prove that Sally had anything to do with me simply because she did it. If you make these kinds of wild charges public, it could be the end of your career, not mine. Don't act like an idiot."

Roger slowly began to calm down. Maybe Sally was lying. She was a bit of an airhead. He ought to throttle the truth out of her. And he knew he suspected George because of that never-explained business with HLV. Now he had the lymphoma virus and new leads on the human colon cancer virus. That young what's-his-name, Charlie something, was coming to show him his results later today. And this time no contaminants. One hint of scandal at this point would bring the goddamn reporters swarming. So he couldn't bring anything up to Musson until he was sure, absolutely sure, of his facts. But he had to get the last word.

"George, I don't like you. We've both been at the FCI for a long time. The others, Abelson, Buchner and Levitt, are out of the picture. You've shaved every corner to stay competitive with me and I've still beaten you. My lab is now twice as large as yours and one way or another, I'm going to see that you are kicked out of here on your sneaky fat ass."

Could the bastard really be thinking what George thought he was? Could he have fixed the site visit scheduled for next week, perhaps plant something in his lab? He'd have to really be careful, return the threat but not show his apprehension.

"Don't you threaten me!" the shorter man's voice rose. "You forget, I'm not without resources, and you're pushing me to the limit. I'll be watching carefully. If I can prove any form of irregularity in any of the scientific review my laboratory undergoes in the next year, Musso will have to explain it to the reporters and it will be your career on the line."

The two men, top cancer researchers, respected scientists, Nobel candidates, stood glaring at each other like small boys battling in a playground over who had more territory. If the air hadn't reeked of the hatred, the scene would be almost comical, the short, pudgy, calmer man glaring up at his still-enraged taller rival. And as Roger stormed out of the room, the audience, listening carefully in the outer office, knew that the Roger and George show was far from over.

Roger charged back across the FIH campus to his lab. The bright sunlight stung his eyes, and that compounded with his racing heart following his confrontation with George, made him feel like he might collapse. How he'd love to destroy the obese little toad! But he'd wait till after he got his Nobel Prize.

It had taken Roger Salla nearly two decades to get where he was now, on the brink of revealing a viral cause for a common human cancer. And then, only then, he would achieve his lifelong goal of fame. Funny, most people who craved recognition went into the arts, something showy that anyone could appreciate. But Salla had chosen virology, and had been sucked into the cancer problem. It wasn't enough for him to contribute something to science and help human suffering. His needs were more down-to-earth.

He wanted fame.

Had the word "nerd" existed in the 1950s, it would have described Roger Salla perfectly. Instead, the kinder of his high school classmates called the skinny kid Poindexter. But Roger didn't really mind. He was just biding his time until college, when he knew his analytical mind could really shine. And shine it did in an era when Sputnik made the American public respect the scientifically gifted, not like today, when people cared more for an IRA than DNA.

Another word that would have fit Salla, had it been invented, was workaholic. Seven day weeks, 18 hour days, were the norm. In his second year at Tufts, he had discovered the world of research and his hours in the library were replaced with hours in the lab. His grades fell ever-so-slightly as he cut his huge lecture classes to spend more time in the microbiology lab.

In graduate school, his familiarity with the ways of scientists paid off. He whizzed through to his Ph.D. in an unprecedented two years, mostly because he latched onto a project that he knew would work, while his fellow grad students floundered about in different labs, trying to decide what they were interested in, but without the talent to zero in on which projects would yield answers in the shortest time possible. That, Salla sensed, was the secret to successful research.

And he was right.

By the time he'd earned his Ph.D., Roger Salla had already published 10 papers. A post-doctoral stint at Harvard over the next three years earned him 16 more and people -- the right people -- were beginning to take notice.

He'd started at the FCI almost two decades ago as a junior scientist with just one technician, and not a very good one at that. Today he was the best known virologist in the world, commanding a laboratory of 30 scientists and more than 100 technicians with an annual budget in excess of $20 million. His lab was not only the largest at the FCI, but by general agreement, the most productive. More than one hundred papers issued forth from within the poster-covered walls each year and Salla saw to it that his name was on the best third of them, at the very least.

Roger had decided sometime during grad school that the person to discover a viral cause of human cancer -- horrible as the idea was -- would earn a Nobel prize. He was now convinced of two things -- that such a virus existed, and that he would be the one to find it. And so he was a man obsessed, a fact known to everyone in the Institute, especially those in his lab. And today the kid they had called Poindexter was now called "Salla, the slave-driver."

It was an accurate assessment.

Roger was sweating profusely in the August heat by the time he got to Building 37, rushing through the gleaming labs to his enormous office. It was a mecca for paper. Piles were everywhere, and only if you got close could you appreciate the incredible organization that took 40 hours a week of attention from a secretary assigned to "paper duty." The pile farthest to the left was reprints, next to it preprints, and next to that, papers nearing final draft stage. Then the piles got a little more ragged, until the one farthest to the right consisted of scrawlings and lists that represented the thoughts of some of the top virologists and cancer researchers in the world. Salla could find any particular paper in just seconds. And if he couldn't, the poor GS-10 on paper duty could look elsewhere for a job.

On a large blackboard in back of the desk, six neatly written names headed six columns. This was where Salla kept track of his senior scientists, directing their every activity. No paper was written, no slide was made, no observation was published without Roger's advice and consent. Some appreciated this close attention, but others felt stifled. It was often joked that the group leaders' bathroom habits should be included on the chart as well, and someone had done just that last April 1. The boss had not been amused.

All the scientists working in the neat laboratories in Building 37 knew they had a single goal -- not anything so lofty as curing cancer, or even understanding it, but to provide the voracious Roger with new data, to churn out a constant stream of material for his presentations at national meetings, anything that would propel him on his chosen path to the coveted Prize.

He was absolute hell to work for. And no one knew this better than Charlie Templeton.

The handsome young scientist stood at Roger's door, suffering obviously from "Salla syndrome." His face ticked, his underarms were soaked, he shifted uneasily from one foot to the other. Templeton had waited for this moment for two years, and he was determined not to screw up. He faced the maddening task of having to present his own, original work as having been inspired by Salla's great leadership.

Actually, in the two years that the young man had spent meticulously looking through colon cancer cell lines for anything resembling a viral particle, he'd spoken to the slave driver only a handful of times. And anytime he'd reported a possible important result, Salla's response was ridicule.

But now Charlie was certain that he had something. Within the last six months, he'd developed a new assay to detect a viral protein, and on rescreening several cell lines, was sure he was on the right track. There was something in there all right. And it was a short step from a viral protein to knabbing the virus itself. He even had the proverbial picture worth a thousand words -- an electron microscope (EM) photograph showing what looked like a virus budding from a cell membrane. How Salla would love to show that one at the next conference! And how Charlie would love to publish this work independently, but he knew there'd be no chance of that. His name would be lost among a dozen or so on the paper in Nature. No one would even know that the work had been really his alone.

But such was life at the FCI. It still beat struggling for grants at the University of North Dakota.

Charlie hardly noticed the admiring stares of the secretary and receptionist as he walked over to Salla's door and knocked. He heard a grunt from within and entered.

Roger was at his corner table writing furiously. Without looking up, he said sharply, "Yes, yes. What is it?" "Dr. Salla, sir, it's time for us to review those preliminary findings on the protein I discussed with you last week. Remember?" he nearly choked.

"Of course I remember. Now, what was that you found again?"

Charlie cleared his throat. "I think I now have confirmatory evidence of the viral protein."

Salla stopped writing and looked up into the frightened face. "Come here Charlie, I want to look at what you have."

The younger man obediently handed his boss the diagrams, tables, gels and EMs and stood back. He knew better than to explain anything to Salla who, despite his reputation as an evil top sergeant, knew more than any other person in the world about viruses. Charlie awaited the inevitable barrage of questions.

Ten minutes passed. A good sign.

"Hey, I think we may have something here."

Charlie held onto the table at about the position of the preprints for support, he was so relieved. And then came the speech.

"But obviously, this work is preliminary and will require a great deal of help from me. I've seen these kinds of observations before, a young scientist who thinks he has the world by the nuts, doing a few experiments, and thinking a new virus is there just for him to discover. But it isn't that easy." He leaned back in his chair and scanned the sheets again.

"I wouldn't have come to you if I wasn't certain I was onto something, Sir." Don't get too defensive now, Charlie.

"You misunderstand. This is fine work. But to verify it, I'm going to have to put a whole research team on this project, screening cell lines and replicating your findings. If they can be replicated."

They would be the other nine names on his paper, Charlie thought.

"And we've got to actually see the virus, this EM budding is good, but not good enough for publication. No matter how many enzyme assays we publish, everyone wants to get a look at the damned thing," Roger barked. He scanned a few moments more. "Yes, yes, there's an interesting lead here. The levels of the protein are extraordinarily high and the consistency of your work is solid." It was the closest to praise that Roger Salla ever gave. "I want you to bring your work to the senior research conference this afternoon and present it to Ivan Gamel and the others. If they agree with my assessment, we will put half the lab on this project and wrap it up in three months."

Charlie's voice was squeaky as he blurted, "But Dr. Salla, I've worked for more than two years on these assays. I would like to finish it and publish it myself. You know how important this work is to me." He knew he had made a mistake even as he uttered the words.

Roger Salla's ugly features twisted into the grotesque Frankenstein monster. He leaned forward and grabbed the small paperweight-like award from the Stibble Foundation as "Outstanding Virologist for 1978" clenching it as if it was a weapon. He cleared his throat, getting ready for his famous bellow. "I know no such thing and what's more, I don't care. What's important to you is of no importance in this matter."

Charlie shrank back, awaiting the onslaught.

"This work is being done in my laboratory and you're working with my resources, you're working under my direction, and all of your thoughts pertaining to research over the past two years have been shaped by working with me. Without my help you wouldn't know an original observation from a horse's ass."

"But sir, you just said..."

Salla was shouting now. "You get the hell back out to the lab, and run these assays over. Be thankful that I allow you to work here -- that I recognize your work."

"Yes sir," the younger man muttered.

"And remember, I want you in here this afternoon to meet with my senior research team, and we're gonna proceed with this project as we do with all the others to come out of this lab -- under my direction, with my resources, and if we verify your preliminary results, I'll report them to the world."

Charlie backed out of the room, his whole body trembling. He felt an embarrassing dampness on his trousers and knew it wasn't sweat. He barely noticed the receptionist patting his back and the secretary bringing him a glass of water as he hurried to get away from his obviously deranged boss as fast as possible.

What a week! Just two days ago he'd given Stephen the latest findings on the lymphoma virus. Instead of hailing his progress, Musso had bitched about why it had taken so long, complaining that he'd barely have time to get it ready to present in the fall. Of course, Roger had wanted to present it himself -- after all, his lab had discovered the damned thing, but he knew that when the paper came out, Stephen's name would be the one recognized by the press, by the world.

Catching the ditsy technician Sally monkeying around with his cultures had scared and enraged him and that shouting match with Trumpey only made it all worse. But now maybe the young Templeton would save him. The kid was a damned fine researcher and far enough below Roger on the FCI ladder and intimidated enough so that he still exerted complete control.

Colon cancer was his baby. Five times the number of lymphoma patients developed colon cancer yearly. Many were productive, influential people. Roger estimated the colon cancer problem solution to be ten times the value of that for lymphoma. Let Musso have some of the lymphoma virus credit if he wanted it so badly. The colon cancer virus, with Templeton's help, would get him the Prize.

CHAPTER 8

THE SHATTERED DREAM

Fall 1956

Rob's mind was already beginning to wander and the lecture had just begun. Law school was a bore. Case after case, principle after principle, resolution after resolution. It all seemed like a game and a repetitious one. Defendant, plaintiff, the system, over and over. Ideally, the system should serve both parties well with true justice as the end point. However, Rob had come to recognize that such was often not the case. So he sat there, listening to the professor drone on about the specifics of Smithers vs. Connecticut. And he couldn't help but think how almost irrelevant the law really was.

But he hadn't always thought that way. Growing up in the massive white mansion in Groton, Connecticut, sheltered from anything remotely resembling controversy or dissatisfaction, Rob Tomasi initially thought nearly everyone came from a household with servants, where all one's needs were automatically met. As a youngster, the toughest decision he had to make was whether to vacation at the family hideaway in the Berkshires or in the summer home on Nantucket (or maybe at the digs of one of his dad's cronies). After all, John Tomasi, Director and Chairman of Chemical Industries Inc., knew everyone of importance in all of New England. And even when he was sent away to prep school he didn't see much of the world, the real world, for his schoolmates came from the same background as he.

Rob was an attractive boy, obviously on his way to more than a six foot frame, well proportioned and muscular. Light brown hair, full and always tousled with deep chestnut eyes reflecting his warmth of personality and quick mental acuity. Friendship, influence and girls came easily to this young man.

That Rob would go from Choate to Harvard law school was never doubted. He was an only child of wealthy, socially, and politically prominent parents, and this was the role chosen for him. His family had spoken of Harvard law for as long as he could remember, and they delighted in his enthusiasm for a career in law and politics. But what his parents didn't know was the real reason why he was now sitting in this stifling classroom.

Rob didn't choose law school to please or appease his parents or anyone else. He went simply because he truly believed that the world was an unjust one, and that perhaps as an attorney and ultimately a politician, he could right some wrongs. But, of course, such thoughts were unpopular in the 50s and he wisely kept them to himself.

Rob grew even more troubled in law school, troubled by his own good fortune at being born rich and by the system of justice that often seemed to serve only those who could afford to use it, twist it, and even abuse it. As he memorized principle after principle, he knew they didn't apply in the real world, not for the blacks, the disadvantaged and the poor. Although he recognized that no perfect system of justice could ever be created, he was struck by the pervasiveness with which injustice intruded into the daily lives of ordinary people.

Towards the end of law school, Rob came to the conclusion that justice was more a political than a legal concept. How else could Nazi Germany have considered mass murder not only "legal" but a solution to a problem? Rob was stimulated by the political process. While a law could perhaps deliver justice on a case by case basis, it was the system politic that really delivered justice in the broader sense. He knew so well from his family and their friends how the political system could be manipulated. Sure, he had used his family's wealth to pay his tuition these past eight years, but soon he'd be on his own to build a reputation in addressing the inequity of justice in the

United States. He would be the one to change the system. He'd need power, but he'd earn it and use it properly. Even if it required an eventual end to his family's "old-boy" network.

As Rob daydreamed through the final days of law school, he became aware of an inner conflict. Yes, he might have to use his family's connections to enter politics and rise so that he could effect a change. A change which could undo the forces that had enabled him to reach his position. He knew that he'd have to keep his ultimate goals quiet, at least for now. Talking of equality, reasonable access, real justice and a responsive and efficient government did not win many votes. Most people cared about a pretty face, a strong voice and emotional appeals. But who knew what the sixties might bring?

So as graduation approached, he knew what he must do -- hold his innermost thoughts private while he positioned himself to change the system. And he knew how to do it -- get himself elected.

1966

The heat was intense, the lights blinding, the noise deafening and the room packed. The newly-elected youthful senator from Connecticut loved it, standing up there before his friends and family, his arm around his stunning wife, Catherine, two handsome children standing in front with his prominent parents beaming at his side. The perfect American family. Rob kissed his wife and walked up to the microphone.

"Ladies and gentlemen. I want to thank all of you for your support and your votes. I know many of you have taken time from your jobs, your families, your recreation to help in this political campaign. I intend to go to Washington and take those issues we have discussed during the last four months directly to the Senate of the United States. Connecticut needs better schools, better roads, better health care, and better educational institutions. We need more jobs and equal opportunity for all. And most importantly, the country needs a more responsive Senate. With your support and with a great deal of conviction and hard work, I hope to represent the state well and have some influence on federal policies in the coming years. You have all worked hard during this campaign. And now it is my turn. I want to thank my family, my friends, my campaign staff, and all of you who have supported me through this election. I will do my best to justify your confidence."

The response was so loud it was almost painful. His wife's beautiful eyes brimmed with tears and her display of emotion was captured by many a photographer. Rob looked out over the sea of party hats and champagne glasses, flowers landing in his already tousled brown hair. A breathless young worker came up and put a strand of beads around his neck and kissed him full on the mouth. Any why not have a good time? Despite his words to the contrary, life wasn't really too bad in Connecticut in the "turbulent" sixties, at least not for the people in attendance at this reception. They all had jobs and their kids were safe at home with their student deferments.

Robert Tomasi was exactly where he wanted to be -- 37 years old and newly elected to the Senate. Sure, his family connections had helped, plus the friends he'd carefully made while practicing law in New Haven. But now he could finally start to do what he had intended all along, make some changes. He fully intended to deliver on every one of his campaign promises. Only a handful of his partying admirers knew anything of Tomasi's real plans. Senator from Connecticut, yes, for now. But Robert Tomasi intended to become, and very well might become, President of the United States.

Fall 1979

"Senator, there are 30 million Americans who are uninsured or underinsured. Senator Bolley wants your support on a new supplement to Medicare which would extend that program to people of all ages and be the basis for a form of federal health insurance."

So ended the presentation of Rob Tomasi's young and eager aide. He was an enthusiast and very socially conscious, a holdover from the decade before. He was thin and angular, had shaved off his beard and his hair was now carefully combed. But, he continued to support programs that might help the disadvantaged, and health care was his major concern. In today's staff meeting, he was again trumpeting a health care initiative for the Senator to consider.

Senator Tomasi rubbed his jaw for a few moments, a sign that he was thinking through his answer. "Well, I think Senator Bolley's proposal is a good one. Like many plans for the uninsured, it is conceptually on target. Unfortunately, like most of these ideas, Senator Bolley hasn't bothered to structure the fiscal support needed to carry out this plan." He paused and looked around at the attentive faces. "I am truly amazed to see people proposing entitlement program after program without regard to how to pay for them. Health care in this country has largely been supported by cross subsidy. The insured and the wealthy pay the hospital costs of the poor, the unemployed and uninsured. I think it is time for government to get serious about this issue and identify specific taxes to carry out programs."

It was no wonder that the young aide was so hyped up about equitable health care, for it was a pet concern of the Senator, a major theme of both his re-election campaigns and of his years in the Senate. He'd even proposed a "pay-your- own-way" tax. And the aides would certainly never forget the reports they had compiled on the health effects of cigarettes and alcohol, and of automobile-accident statistics, to prepare the Senator's proposals of steep taxes on these three commodities that contributed so heavily to heath care costs. The logic was obvious. Tax alcohol and cigarettes to pay for their detrimental effects on health. Tax automobile sales and gasoline to pay for the accident related health costs. Very business like. Use the commodity and pay for its effects on society. But despite the team's best efforts, none of Tomasi's innovative proposals had become law. And they all knew why -- special interests. The tobacco lobby, the liquor lobby and the automobile and petroleum lobbies. It seemed that for every new initiative in the United States Senate, there was a lobby both for and against it. And the popular, well-meaning Senator from Connecticut realized that he could propose, but not effectuate, innovation.

Fall 1980

Maintaining an appropriate social life in two communities for an extremely popular young senator was difficult at any time but in a Presidential election year, it was nearly impossible. Good thing tonight's dinner was only for twelve. Although the servants did all the work and did it well, Catherine felt that she had to be around, making sure everything was ready on time and in the right place. After thirteen years in Washington she knew well the general purpose of these dinners and this one was no exception -- bring together the right group of people, and a particular legislative initiative would receive the right push.

Catherine was downstairs fussing with the flowers and Rob was still in the shower when the doorbell rang. Catherine knew who it was, for Senator Daniels was always the first to arrive so he could get at the food first. And her suspicions were confirmed when she caught a whiff of musky perfume. She often wondered whether the Senator intentionally sought women who reeked of perfume or required them to douse themselves once he dated them. The gruff old guy had been separated from his wife for several years now and his choice of women was often a source of entertainment at Washington parties. Tonight was no exception.

"Well, Senator, how are you tonight?" Catherine inquired as she graciously accepted the flowers handed to her by the short, stocky man.

"Well, I guess I'm okay, M'am, although it seems difficult to get through some of the crazy things that are happening in Washington these days. Oh, may I introduce Miss Tricia Megan -- such a pretty little thing," he cooed as he patted her on the rear.

It Catherine hadn't already been so used to this behavior she might have been embarrassed for the young woman, who didn't seem to mind being treated like a prize show animal. She was quite beautiful with the stature of a fashion model. It looked sort of funny next to the Senator who resembled an old bullfrog. He weighed close to 250 pounds at 5 feet 6 inches. His dark eyes were hard to follow as they flitted from woman to woman between puffy, globelike lids. Senator Daniels was not very attractive (except, perhaps to a lady frog), but his chairmanship of the Senate Foreign Relations Committee made him a popular and powerful man in Washington. Not surprisingly, exquisite women flocked to his chubby side. But he was, Catherine had to admit, a nice person and fun to have at a party.

No sooner had Catherine ushered Senator Daniels and his companion into the spacious living room and showed them the hors d'ouvres when the bell rang again, and she was caught up in the back and forth game of being the perfect Washington hostess. Good thing she had training from her mother-in-law. Finally, Rob made his entrance and the party broke up into small groups.

As always, the children made their requisite, adorable goodnight visit, the five-course dinner went off without a hitch, dessert was chocolaty perfection and afterwards, the little groups reconvened in the living room for coffee and liqueur. Except for the host, Senator Daniels and John Bixley, who had escaped to the den with glasses of brandy. Those in the larger room seemed to realize the import of the discussion going on in the den and patiently continued their banter about the coming presidential contest between the peanut farmer's vice president and the actor.

The mood was intense in the den. Bixley started things rolling.

"There's no question Rob, you must start considering now when you will declare yourself for '84. It's never too soon." As Carter's Chief of Staff, John Bixley was a man who could say this with some conviction.

"Yes, you have a real constituency out there, and it includes the President. The press loves you and 1984 is only four years away," Daniels agreed. Both men had been trying to coax Tomasi into making his private aspirations more public. The current race had been assessed by these men. Mondale's chances were slim to none. They wanted to discount their loss with a real winner for 1984. They knew they had the full support of the Tomasi clan. Now all they had to do was convince Rob himself. They suspected they were getting close.

Rob sat back and absorbed his colleagues' compliments like a sponge, stroking his jaw. He was growing excited. Maybe the time really was coming, perhaps when the post-election excitement died down. As he looked around at his elegant surroundings, he thought once against his innermost commitments to all the people who he honestly thought he could help. Yes, the time was right.

God, he was tired. One legislative session after another, power breakfasts, influence lunches, endless dinners and meetings with the press. Maybe it was just the excitement of last night's talk with Bixley and Daniels, the realization that he'd start actively seeking the presidency soon. But why on earth was it all so exhausting? He was only 50 and looked ten years younger. He was certainly no newcomer to politics or the pace of Washington life. He just didn't seem able to keep his energy up.

Rob sat back at his desk reading a report prepared by one of his aides. Soon deep in thought his hand passed absently over the angle of his jaw. But this time, instead of enabling him to concentrate, his hand motion distracted him and he put the report down, tracing his fingers over the curve in his jaw again. Yes, there was definitely something new there. That was odd, it almost felt like a small lump. Swollen glands? But he didn't have a sore throat or even a fever or cold. He was just a little tired, that's all.

But even as his consciousness denied what his fingers felt and alarm sounded somewhere deep within him. Healthy people didn't get lumps. Anywhere. He knew he'd have to get it checked out -- quickly and quietly. He'd wait until next week, back in Connecticut.

Three weeks later the truth was known to everyone. Who could miss it with "Senator Tomasi has cancer" blaring forth from the New York Times, the Boston Globe and of course, People magazine. So much for privacy. But he had expected it. He was the golden boy of politics, young, attractive, vibrant and bright, acceptable to most factions of the Democratic party and a Presidential hopeful for '84 or '88. But "the big C" put a stop to his plans.

It all seemed to have happened quickly although Rob realized that he'd been run down and had trouble sleeping for several months. Maybe it was his doctor's forthright manner that had forced him to face up to his situation so abruptly. After the biopsy and follow-up tests, he didn't waste any time at all on chitchat.

"Senator, I'll be blunt. You have cancer."

"Yes, that certainly is blunt. Go on," Roger muttered.

"It's a lymphoma but a kind that is very treatable with chemotherapy and may go on for a very long period of time. However, it is not curable. You'll need some radiation and perhaps some chemotherapy in the short term, but in the long term, this thing is going to change your future plans."

Fortunately, Rob was used to the doctor's approach and he had more or less guessed the nature of his illness, the source of his fatigue. A quick look through some medical books had confirmed his suspicions. But what he didn't know was where to go from here.

"Thank you doctor. Well, I guess I'll just have to decide what to do. Should I go to an oncologist here in Connecticut or should I go to my local cancer center? My wife suggested getting into a research program but should I contact Yale first, seek advice at Sloan Kettering, or go straight to the FCI? Where do I start?" he asked in a voice that he didn't realize was shaking.

"Well, Senator, for the short term it really doesn't matter. You can get radiation and chemotherapy right here and it will probably be effective for a while. But for the longer term, you're absolutely right. My advice is to get involved in research. Especially considering your type of disease."

"What do you mean? Is one type better than another?"

"In a way, yes. Your form of lymphoma has been of real interest to researchers, to immunologists at Stanford and the FCI. There is some possibility that antibodies can be made to counteract your condition. It's being done on an experimental basis now. Yes, I think you should look into that technology."

"What was that? Antiwhat? Aren't antibodies drugs to fight infection? What has that got to do with cancer?"

"You're thinking of antibiotics. Antibodies are proteins made by the immune system. They protect the body by recognizing and attacking substances and cells that don't belong there, like viruses or cancer cells."

"But if they're made by the immune system, how can the FCI get a hold of them?"

"Well, it's kind of complicated. Part of a new technology in which researchers grow huge amounts of antibodies that are directed against a particular patient's tumor cells. It's called monoclonal antibody technology. Here, I'll write it down," the doctor said as he reached for a prescription pad.

"But isn't that kind of expensive? I mean, all that effort to knab one guy's tumor?"

"You're damn right. These antibodies are tough to make. By some estimates they may cost as much as $100,000 per patient and take a year to perfect. Even then there's no guarantee they will work."

"But how do people get this treatment? I mean, who gets into the research studies?"

The doctor was silent for a few moments. "Well, people apply. If they meet certain conditions -- have the type of cancer being studied and have tried traditional routes of treatment, are otherwise healthy -- they might be selected."

"Okay, how do I get started?"

"Well, the first step is to call the FCI, or better yet, I'd have someone in oncology at Yale do it. Then you apply, get on a list. But..."

"But what?" Rob interrupted.

"Well, you really don't have to go that route."

"What do you mean?"

"Senator, you're an important person. God, you could have been our next President! You're not exactly Joe Blow with a lump in the neck. And you've supported legislation that has helped the FCI. You've made a real investment in the system. Now is the time to ask for a fair return."

"What are you saying?"

"How much more blunt need I be? Use your influence, man. It could very well save your life. You can't just sign up at a company, plunk down some money, and have them churn out "magic bullets" to cure your cancer. Maybe someday that'll be possible, but unless you use your influence now, you won't be around to take advantage of it. The answer's in research, and that means getting into an FCI clinical trial or perhaps setting up some sort of grant to get a university lab to make your antibodies. Do it! Anyone in your position would."

What about the 99% of the population not in his position? But he'd never be able to help the millions out there if he didn't get these damn antibodies. The irony of the situation struck full force as Rob thanked the doctor and walked out of the office. He actually chuckled as he walked past the receptionist, who glanced with some concern at the man whom she knew had just been given a devastating diagnosis.

Rob walked through the chilly streets without even buttoning his overcoat, immune to the cold as he thought over his predicament. He walked for miles, deep in thought. Since freshman year in college he had vowed to rise through the political system until he could really do something to bring equality to all people. And now, to obtain that position, he was being forced by an ominous thing growing, out of control, in his neck to use that very influence to buy his own life, in a way not many people could. He would need to use the system he aspired to change to search for a cure. Of course, it was all so that he could help others less fortunate -- the ends justify the means and all that. But it still ate at him.

Just like a cancer.

CHAPTER 9

TELEPHONE RESEARCH

Fall 1975

Nurse Kelly jumped with such a start that she almost upset the medicine tray. Again. By now she should be used to it. But she was only a second year nurse on the oncology ward, and even the veterans said that the gut-wrenching screams from Room 104 were worse than usual. Far worse.

In spite of codeine, Demerol and methadone by mouth, plus a morphine sulfate intravenous drip, Sam Luria continued to shriek in agony from time to time. It wasn't that he was a sissy - he was clearly in tremendous pain. A thin, good-looking, urbane middle-aged man, Sam had been in the hospital six days, and the doctors still didn't know precisely what was wrong with him. He had been transferred from an outlying hospital near Savannah, where his physicians had been unable to diagnose the problem. But it was obvious to all that he was a very sick man indeed.

The pain centered in his back, and it came in short bursts. The nurses could tell when he was about to experience another attack, because he'd clench his fists, then curl up into a fetal position, the only way he could stay reasonably comfortable. Only with huge doses of narcotics would his muscles begin to relax, and he could fall asleep.

Sam was such a lovable guy, despite a faint reek of garlic from food specially prepared outside the hospital. The nurses took special interest in him, and all were concerned about his unremitting pain and the lack of a definitive diagnosis. Nurse Kelly knew that x-rays of the area hadn't told the doctors a thing, but that a bone scan showed a suspicious increase in activity in the lumbar spine. And there was a telltale increase of a certain protein in the blood. A bone marrow was scheduled for tomorrow. She suspected what it might show, given the bone pain and elevated protein. She liked to try to diagnose her patients. And this time, unhappily, she was right. The doctors also suspected multiple myeloma, a cancer of the bone and bone marrow in which excess antibody protein is produced and secreted into the bloodstream. The searing bone pain and muscle spasms echoed the weakening tissue. But none of the staff, doctors or nurses, had ever seen, or heard, the kind of pain that Sam Luria was experiencing.

She left her medicine tray and rushed in to comfort the patient. His face was contorted from the blinding paroxysms of pain, his temples pounding, his hands frantically grappling the bedrails. Between bouts he'd told her that the pain was like a white hot knife twisting slowly inside, coming from the lower mid back and shooting out through his abdomen and down into both testicles, obliterating all thought and control. And this looked like a bad attack.

"Please, please, give me more medicine," he cried. "Hurry, I've got to have some relief from this hell."

Nurse Kelly squeezed Mr. Luria's shoulder. "It's not time for your medication, but let me turn up the morphine drip. I'll call the doctor. I'm sure he will agree to the faster drip. I just can't bear to see you wait until I reach him on his beeper," she said as she reached over to open up the control knobs on the drug monitoring device by three notches. The patient squinted at her intently. "There, you'll feel a difference in a few minutes. Now, you try to relax. I'm going to the nurse's station to call him. I'll be back in a few minutes."

Still curled up like a fetus, Sam looked up at the bottle and the slowly-dripping medicine and waited for the morphine to take effect. Goddamit, he was an addict already! Who the hell cared, he just couldn't stand the pain. And if they didn't do something, know something soon, he'd try to reach up and change those controls himself, turn it all the way up. That would end the pain once and for all.

Soon his mind grew hazy and confused, an increasingly familiar but still odd sensation. He mentally resisted the darkness trying to engulf him to reach the pleasure the morphine would soon bring. The pain ebbed into the background as his mind seemed to separate itself from his body and float somewhere beyond his reach. Past, present and future seemed to merge as wildly colored, three-dimensional images passed before his eyes. It was as if a canvas of his life stretched before him, and he had the power to paint whatever scenes he wished. If only he could take pictures of such incredible beauty! He tried to put the pictures into some sort of logical sequence, but no matter how exquisite the images, they all ran together in the blinding pain.

It seemed as if the pain had been present for years, but in fact, this whole illness, whatever it was, had started barely six weeks ago, in a healthy man, with a sudden onset of low back pain. To the doctors in Savannah, it was a mystery. They thought it was all in his head. And after a psychiatric consultation, Sam began to understand how the almighty doctors thought. If they didn't understand a direct physical cause for pain, they assumed it was psychosomatic. Next stop, a shrink to help the poor patient understand that his symptoms weren't as severe as he thought they were.

The meeting with the psychiatrist was a joke. Sam had brought with him the stereotype of the long bearded, fat-bellied shrink. And sure enough, the doctor, who fit the preconceived bill precisely, had plopped down into a chair and started to babble about sensation and perception and degrees of pain and, by the way, what were your mother and father like? Even in his drug-induced haze, Sam almost laughed aloud as he envisioned the hairy faced, pompous bastard floating by, legs crossed and gloating with pleasure at the tortured soul before him.

Sam had had the sense to get himself out of Savannah and into the university hospital at Mallory. A seat of higher learning, as the college catalogs say. Surely these doctors could figure out what was wrong and fix him up. And they'd realize that it was in his back, not his head.

The haze was beginning to clear, and an increasing part of Sam's consciousness returned to the problems of the present. He was worried about his restaurant, his wife, his children, for all of them were inseparable in his mind. They had lived in Savannah for 30 years, and Sam was the best known Greek restauranteur in the mid South. "The Golden Lamb" was an incredibly successful business, and a major part of that success was due to Sam's finesse on the phone.

In fact, the telephone was practically an extension of his body, because he was rarely without it. He was famous for dispensing with bills, contracts and letters - if it couldn't be done over the phone, Sam Luria wouldn't do it. Sam was a man of his word. He was known all over the South as a man who was always reachable by phone. And indeed, the calls came in 24 hours a day.

"Sam, can you help me with a dinner party for eight?"

"Sam, can you set up a party for 52 for my birthday?"

"Sam, how about an intimate corner for my new girlfriend?"

And Sam the phone man was always ready to serve, because he was a connoisseur of human behavior, and had set up his restaurant to suit human needs. So he offered quiet corners for the discreet, large rooms for the parties, great service, and always, the very best food.

It was a family business. On the side of Sam that wasn't permanently affixed to a telephone was his wife, who watched over the kitchen like a hawk. His children, cousins, and nieces and nephews all worked in the restaurant. Sam felt like Alexander the Great when he could watch his loved ones scamper about, carrying trays loaded with souvlaki and gyros and baklava as he planned even more parties on the phone.

But he didn't feel much like Alexander the Great now. The pain was sneaking up on him again as the morphine response leveled off, and his mind pulled completely back to the present. What the hell was causing the awful pain in his back? Was it a broken bone? But, then why were all these cancer specialists poking at him? He could feel the raw fear rise up out of his gut, like fumes of acid creeping up his chest and bursting out of his mouth. A still nameless fear. He had only to wait for the doctors to confirm it.

It was a beautiful day in Atlanta. The birds were chirping outside Mallory University Hospital, the sun was so bright it hurt the eyes, and the sky was a clear blue. Low humidity and a light breeze brought out the girlfriends and picnic baskets. It was a beautiful day for everyone but Sam Luria.

His physician had just left Room 104. Sam had been right, as patients generally are. He had cancer, and it was not curable. A form of cancer called multiple myeloma. He had gone through the usual physician's speech, telling him what the disease was, what it meant, what the outlook was, what kinds of problems he was likely to have, what kinds of treatments might be of benefit.

Most patients in such circumstances are in a state of shock, hearing little beyond the initial use of the dreaded word "cancer". But Sam had a mind that was different from most. The same mind that enabled him to run one of the finest restaurants in the country was instantly activated, like a computer cataloging information as he assembled it into a logical order and planned ahead. Just as his understanding of people was the key to his success in the restaurant business, his thorough understanding of his disease would be the way to beat it. And beat it he would.

Number one, it was called multiple myeloma. Number two, the cause was unknown. Number three, there was short term treatment that would work for months or maybe if he was lucky, years, but ultimately he would suffer weakened, broken bones, unremitting pain, kidney failure and a bedridden existence. Those were the facts.

On the other hand, his doctor had been somewhat encouraging, more so than Sam had expected. He filed away the names of the drugs as the doctor droned on.

"Some patients take treatment and stabilize," he said. "I've seen myeloma patients take Alkeran and Prednisone for years, and if they don't get into bone marrow reserve problems and their blood counts stay fairly normal, this drug combination can hold the disease at bay for a long time. Other patients manifest what we call 'burnt out myeloma'."

"That sounds ominous," Sam interjected.

"Not really. The patient, after receiving chemotherapy for years, still has pain with an elevated blood protein. Then, for reasons unclear to us, he or she simply stabilizes, and often for a long period of time. Treatment can be held and the patient may be pain free. They're unusual, but your best shot is to start on the two drugs and hope you're one of the fortunate few. As you can probably see, we really don't know too much about this disease."

"Except that I have it."

"Unfortunately, yes."

The doctor was muttering something about rounds, trying gracefully to exit, but Sam's mind was already quite far away. His gaze was on the one thing that could help, come to his aid and initiate his search for a cure - the telephone.

No, it just wouldn't do. He'd need at least three separate numbers, for when the researchers he would soon begin to contact had to get back to him, they musn't face a busy signal. And of course he'd need someone to monitor the phones when he was down in the medical library, which he hoped he could do as soon as they got his pain under some sort of control. The job before Sam Luria was enormous, far worse than planning an eight course banquet for 100 daily for years.

His job was no less than to call every serious researcher in the country, perhaps the world, knowledgeable about this multiple myeloma. Every major university oncologist. He needed to get into and avail himself of the resources of the Federal Cancer Institute. He must get to the journals and read and read and read, and then use a computer to compile and sort out all the facts. He needed no pen or paper to form his plan, as it created itself in his feverish mind.

He knew how to begin the search. He'd fight his cancer on the phone.

CHAPTER 10

USING THE SYSTEM

<u>1968</u>

Stanley Lizzard was in his least favorite place - a packed elevator destined for the 17th floor of Cornell Medical Center. There must have been nearly two dozen people crammed in like so many sardines, a combination of doctors, nurses, maintenance workers and patients, and several emitted the sour odor of missed baths. One man in the back had the nerve to light a cigarette - something that should be punishable by death, Stanley thought. And a stout woman in front had very obviously consumed a rather foul smelling anchovy sandwich for lunch.

The stench and overcrowding made Stanley panicky and sick to his stomach. Somehow crowded situations always reminded him of his parents' three-room tenement in New York City. He'd been stuffed into a stifling room with two brothers and two sisters. With heat in the winter a rarity, the nightly bath down the hall between two apartments was often foregone. Frequently, the young Stanley would crawl out onto the fire escape in the middle of the night just for breathing space. No wonder he was a claustrophobic adult!

He wished he could crawl out somewhere now, as he fought back the impulse to scream and throttle the smoker and Miss Fish-breath. He couldn't stand it, he simply had to get out. So pushing past a fat lady, probably a hypothyroidism case, he muttered "excuse me" and punched the button for the 10th floor. Walking seven flights was infinitely better than suffocating. And the second the elevator doors opened, Stanley bolted, landing with his hands on a dusty windowsill littered with dead insects. The panic began to subside. He gazed down at the city and realized once again how much he detested it - its overcrowding, its filth, its impersonality, the rudeness and coldness of its people. Thank God in only six more months he could leave it all behind!

Stanley was headed for no less than the prestigious Federal Cancer Institute. He'd fought long and hard to get his appointment as a clinical associate. In this era of the Vietnam "conflict", every smart physician on the East Coast was trying to get into the FCI and the Public Health Service (PHS). No wonder the armed services called the PHS the "yellow berets".

The young doctor knew that a trip to Vietnam would be the end for him. Even if the enemy didn't get him, the viruses, bacteria, contaminated drinking water and poor sanitary conditions there surely would. If he couldn't stand the overcrowding of an elevator in a supposedly sophisticated city, how would he fare crammed aboard a military transport, or sharing barracks, or wedged into a hole in the ground? He felt the familiar panicky nausea just at the thought. Besides his physical health, he knew a tour in Vietnam would spell the end of his career. So he'd done all he could to escape, and it had worked.

In 1968, a young and healthy physician had but a few ways to get out of the draft. He could go to Canada. He could commit suicide. Or, he could join the PHS. If he was lucky, he could continue with some research in his area of interest. If he was unlucky, he was stuck on an Indian Reservation in Arizona. Either was considerably better than a case of jungle rot in Southeast Asia.

The FCI would be heaven, Stanley knew. Gleaming white laboratories instead of foul-smelling, always complaining patients. If only he could get through the rest of his residency in this pit and not blow up under the stress, he'd have the chance to do the research he really ached for, the opportunity of a lifetime, at the FCI. Civilization.

Stanley was a man not well understood by anyone who knew him, and no one could claim to be really close to him. He was not married, in fact never seemed to have a girlfriend, never seemed to have any friends at all. Yet he had been a straight A student, seemingly calm and friendly. He was quite good-looking, tall and dark with an athletic build, which was more genetics than work because he worried too much about getting injured to exercise. Women would often turn to look at him - his doctor's whites accentuated his swarthy attractiveness, but he never looked back. No one, not his professors or peers, had even a glimpse of the constant churning that was going on beneath his skin. Granted, Vietnam was certainly something to worry about. But Stanley always had something to worry about.

That, too probably stemmed from his childhood. When he wasn't fleeing to the fire escape, he was often at the bottom of a pile of kids who were pummeling him. He never really understood why he was always picked on, but he'd grown up used to violence and abuse. Part of it was his heritage, his name pronounced Liz-zard, all the bullies at school berated him with Stanley the Lizard. If he complained to his parents, they'd pick on him too, accusing him of being a coward and a sissy. His father would beat him and, at the same time, tell him to stop crying. "Be a man!" he would scream. So he'd learned. He'd learned to suppress his feelings and carry them inside so no one would know he was hurting. He'd never let feelings keep him from reaching goals. And his goal was to be on top of that pile. If there was kicking to be done, Stanley would be the kicker, not the kickee!

January 1980

The Atlanta Convention Center was packed. It was the annual meeting of the American Society of Clinical Oncology (ASCO). And as usual, everyone who was anyone in cancer research and treatment was there. Today, at 9:00 a.m., the highly-respected FCI researcher Dr. Stanley Lizzard would present his most recent findings on the ARA-C membrane transport system. The moderator was shuffling some papers, and the introduction began.

"Ladies and gentleman, as our keynote speaker, I would like to introduce Dr. Stanley Lizzard. As most of you know, Dr. Lizzard has published more than 220 papers in the medical literature, and has had quite an illustrious career with the FCI. Over the last five years, as chief of the Laboratory of Clinical Drug Development, he has played a major role in bringing not less than seven anticancer drugs to our clinical practices. The insight provided by his work has allowed those of you who are medical oncologists to deliver anticancer drugs in a safe and effective manner. Much of the understanding of how to use these drugs has come from Dr. Lizzard and his colleagues."

Applause.

"As a specific example of his insightful and brilliant work, Dr. Lizzard has published several major papers on cell membrane transport systems for drugs. Perhaps the one for which he is best known is the classic paper in the "Proceedings of the National Academy of Science" describing the enzyme system which transports cytosine araboniside (ARA-C) from the cell surface to its active site internally. Dr. Lizzard believes the principles learned from dissecting this transport system may allow us to better characterize tumor cell sensitivity and resistance. I am pleased to introduce Dr. Lizzard. His presentation is entitled, "ARA-C Transport System: A Broadly Applicable Model."

The ovation was strong, some in the front rows standing as the handsome young cancer researcher made his way to the podium. Dr. Lizzard had become a popular member of the cancer research establishment, and was a major proponent of chemotherapy drug development as the best hope for cancer control. He had been at the FCI for 12 years, and during that time had risen from clinical associate to laboratory chief. Much of that rise was well deserved, earned by his ability to focus his research project and publish his results. But much of it was due to his relationship with Stephen Musso, who had taken quite a liking to him. When Stephen was chief of the medicine branch, Stanley was one of his boys. And with each step that Stephen took, Stanley was a half-step behind. As Stephen's laboratory and clinical service became larger, so did Stanley's. And when Stephen became head of cancer therapy, Stanley became a laboratory chief. Now there were rumors that Stephen might soon become director of all of FCI. If so, everyone expected Stanley to follow in his footsteps as director of cancer therapy.

The crowd quieted and settled down as Stanley cleared his throat.

"Ladies and gentlemen, it is indeed a pleasure to present the Joseph and Hilda Greenspan Lecture before ASCO. Many of you are in the practice of oncology and you use anticancer drugs daily. What I am going to tell you today represents my own view of one transport system for one drug. However, I would like to suggest that the principles from this transport system are generally applicable across all of our current anticancer drugs and many that we now have in development at the FCI. I believe that a firm understanding of these transport systems will allow us to define why some cells are sensitive and how they become resistant. Once we understand the mechanisms of resistance, it's only a short step away from developing more curative regimens for the drug treatment of cancer."

He paused for a moment. Stephen Musso, seated with Sam Fish on the front row, beamed.

"There are many clues as to how to proceed. Today I will illustrate methods by which one model membrane transport system can be manipulated to increase the sensitivity of cells to ARA-C, and other methods that may help avoid resistance to this important drug. I think you will be able to see the general applications in your practice."

As Stanley spoke, the audience's attention was firmly fixed on the podium. Unlike the claustrophobia he felt in his childhood bedroom and in the Cornell elevator, he felt open and expansive in front of a large audience. He had developed into a talented speaker, and knew how his carefully chosen, almost lyrical words could hold a group's attention. He was second only to Musso in his ability to both entertain and manipulate through the spoken word. It was a gift, and he knew it.

At the back of the room, two other eminent scientists, well aware of Stanley's persuasive capabilities, were whispering. Drs. Adrian Free and Thomas Frederick were growing quite disturbed over the continuing trumpeting of membrane transport systems as the major method to understand drug activity and resistance. Certainly any clear-thinking scientist would realize that a problem had to be tackled from more than one angle. But then again, the honchos at the FCI were anything but clear-thinking, unless it concerned their particular narrow goals.

The F&F twins had had illustrious careers at the FCI. They had departed government in anger, but each had carved a successful career in university research. And both knew intimately the dangerous duo of scientific politics and government bureaucracy. Dr. Lizzard's campaign looked hauntingly familiar, the constant reiteration that there was one major route to success, the appeals for more and more public money for drug development, funds to understand drug resistance, yet more support to develop model systems on membrane transport of anticancer agents. Sure it was important, but so were many other approaches.

What it all translated into was more money for Stephen Musso, and by way of association, Stanley Lizzard.

Although it pained each of them, the F&F twins inevitably ended up discussing FCI politics whenever they met at meetings such as this one.

"Tom, I just can't stand it anymore, even though I'm away from it," said Adrian. "The problems of cancer biology are so much more diverse than drug resistance based on membrane transport systems. There needs to be more flexibility in the federal grants system to provide for other approaches. Can't these bozos see that?"

"Of course they see it, but they choose to ignore it," retorted his equally frustrated colleague. "But you know the system as well as I. Sure, there are a series of rules and regulations that allows the bureaucracy to function, but the real way it works is through the personal agendas of the people in charge. You remember, when the director of the FCI was an epidemiologist, epidemiology funding was king. When the director's baby was chemical carcinogenesis, that was #1, and when cancer prevention rose to the top, everybody and his brother studied cancer prevention. Now it's drug resistance and virology, and it's reflected in the grants program and the emphasis on contract funding. The FCI sets up the review groups to manipulate and program the results. It's the same old story, it just seems more blatant to us since we were victims of the system. Musso and that slimy Lizzard, and to some extent Roger Salla, have put the taxpayers' one billion dollar purse in their back pocket, and they're using it to fund their own interests."

"Well Tom, you old radical! Although your viewpoint is a bit polar, it does seem to be worse since we left, the lack of diversity I mean. The "Musso family" is gradually dominating every phase of work, and it's damn difficult, almost impossible, for someone with an original idea, different from theirs, to get a government grant."

"What do you mean polar? It's the damn truth."

They were interrupted by some vehement "sshhs" from their neighboring listeners, who were held in rapt attention by the magical voice of Stanley Lizzard. They hastily excused themselves and headed out for the hallway to continue their exchange.

February 2, 1980

Stanley was in his overcrowded office in conference with two of his section chiefs. They were presenting some recent data on tumor cell resistance to ARA-C when the door burst open, and Stanley's secretary, a rather plump, redheaded GS- 11, burst in.

"Sorry to interrupt. Have you heard the news? Dr. Musso has just been named FCI director!"

The three scientists stood and whooped. They knew Poldosky had resigned, and it had been rumored for weeks that Musso was next in line. Of the three, Stanley appeared the least excited, probably because he had been expecting this. He knew the process well. Although Stephen never revealed the details of his manipulations to any of his associates, Stanley had a good idea of what had transpired. It was vintage Musso. A little investigation, a little discussion, a thinly veiled threat, usually of a personal nature, and another scientist moves on to a "better" opportunity. With each carefully planned manipulation, Stephen's power base grows, and "his family" is enhanced. It pleased Stanley, for he knew he was Stephen's favored "son".

But now Stephen had really, finally done it. He'd reached the pinnacle, the director. Stanley's excitement mounted as he recalled a discussion he'd had with Stephen after his ASCO presentation in Atlanta. Once Stephen had secured the directorship, he'd promised, Stanley would be made director of the division of therapy. And so the pattern of Stanley following in Stephen's footsteps would continue, all the way to the top.

"Yippee!," yelled Tony South, quite uncharacteristically. "That means less money for carcinogenesis from Dr. Poldosky, and more money for drug development from Dr. Musso."

"Absolutely," chortled his colleague. "Now all we have to do is get Stanley here to replace Musso, and both of our laboratories can be doubled. Man, have I got some projects that need attention. Stanley, when do you think you'll hear from Stephen?"

"Hold on a minute," cautioned Stanley. "Don't you think you're being a bit premature, not to mention juvenile? I'm still chief of this laboratory. The resources I have are the same as they were five minutes ago, and your labs haven't suddenly doubled. Let's wait until Stephen is solid in his job and handing out opportunities before we get excited."

"But ..." they sputtered at the same time, unable to hold their excitement in check. And neither could their boss.

"Well, I guess it wouldn't hurt to begin planning the expansion of our horizons," Stanley thought out loud. "For example, I think now is the time for your interest in the action of viruses on cell membranes to be better tied to Tony's interest in the mechanisms of cell resistance at the membrane level. If certain events come to pass, as I suspect they will, I plan to create a new task force for the two of you to co-chair in an attempt to determine what role viruses may have in altering transport membrane systems for anticancer drugs. As you know, Roger Salla has more and more evidence that viruses are involved in causing cancer. It may be that they're involved not only in causing it, but also contribute to drug resistance. I'm very interested in this virus business, and the relationship to drug resistance."

"But why? Shouldn't we be turning towards new drug discovery, rather than picking apart the mechanisms of resistance to existing drugs?" asked Tony.

"Use your head. If drugs are developed to inhibit viruses, all of us may have less research to do in the future. However, if we can make a strong story for viruses altering membranes and affecting drug resistance, we'll have decades more work to do in the laboratory to better define this phenomenon. And don't forget, Stephen is absolutely committed to Roger. We must support his work."

Both looked a little confused, but soon came around to their boss' way of seeing things. Stanley noted their momentary hesitation, then added, "Don't worry boys. I can assure you of one thing. If I'm given a shot in the arm by Stephen, both of you will get a jolt too." He broke into a grin and shook both their hands.

And so 1980 started out fine indeed for those involved in the drug research program at the FCI. Their champion had just been made director. His chief henchman was appointed to lead cancer therapy. With the two major proponents of drug development safely in place, the future looked bright, and everyone was lining up for their piece of the pie - the pharmaceutical companies, the universities with drug development laboratories, the drug toxicology contract programs, the chemical screening programs, and all the selected university investigators who worked in the highly regulated system of testing new drugs in patients. Even the FDA was pleased. Drug development and testing was well standardized. Their horizons were clear. Across the nation new grant applications, slanted towards drug development, were rapidly but carefully prepared, and at the FCI, new committees formed seemingly overnight as old boy networks readjusted to fit the expanded paradigm. Enthusiasm ran high.

And as was always the case, each time the kingdom changed hands, the rules changed. And cancer research according to Stephen Musso meant drug development. In the back rooms of universities, in the conference halls at meetings, over dinners, by telephone, the various constituencies of the FCI drug development program began to work. It wasn't always clean, but it was efficient. A phone call here, a paper sent there, a carefully chosen committee, a grant given special favors, a little influence on this, and an implied threat on that.

Musso's reign had begun.

CHAPTER 11

BACK TO THE UNIVERSITY

July 5, 1970

"Robert, give me a hand. I've got to get these boxes upstairs."

He was sweating profusely. Midsummer in Washington was pure hell. He and Mary Margaret had arrived in a U-haul truck with an old Ford in tow. With one child here and another on the way, they had hoped to find a small house, but the prices were astronomical, far beyond their means. So they ended up in an efficiency apartment. It was in a good location, walking distance from the FIH Clinical Center, but it was tiny and needed lots of fixing up. But the landlord seemed pleasant, even gave them the supplies to paint and clean if they would do the work. Fortunately, both he and Mary Margaret were good at that sort of thing, and they worked away as the baby slept peacefully, despite the heat.

"O.K. Let me get these things upstairs, and then we can break for lunch."

In spite of the labor, the sweat, and the unending heat, Robert felt more invigorated than he ever had before. This was his chance to really get into the research that he had so long admired. He was at the Federal Cancer Institute to study, to learn, and to work with physicians and scientists he had read about, but whom he had never had the opportunity to meet or get to know. He'd actually work with the likes of Drs. Free and Frederick, and maybe even talk to Dr. Stephen Musso.

He couldn't wait to get started.

The ward was nearly deserted. The only motion was the ghostlike flitting of the few nurses between the rooms, from which an occasional whine or groan would emerge. The air seemed to have an ambiance of overwhelming despair. Coming to this particular ward was the only part of being an FCI oncologist that Robert dreaded.

Tonight he had been called to start an intravenous (IV) on a patient who had leukemia. So what was the problem? He started IVs on cancer patients all the time. In fact, his primary task at the FCI, revered research establishment, seemed to be to start IVs. The Institute used physicians-in- training to draw blood, start IVs and even to empty bedpans. This was a good way, it was thought, to train them to be clinical scientists. Anyway, he didn't mind starting IVs on the adult floor. In every respect, he wanted to do everything that needed to be done to care for a cancer patient, and if this was part of the job, he meant to do it and do it right. But tonight he'd been called down to the third floor, and that was a different story altogether.

The third floor was the pediatric ward. Robert was an adult oncologist, but at the FCI, the adult oncologists covered for the pediatric oncologists at night. And when the IV went bad, whoever was on call had to perform.

Robert smelled the familiar odor of illness as he entered the room. The pale, small boy lying in the bed had diarrhea. The chart said he was six, but he looked no more than four. He had suffered from leukemia for more than two years, and he was one of the potential "cures" the newspaper reporters write about. Sure, his leukemia was in complete remission. But what the reports often left out was that the "cure" came at a terrible price, for he was still on toxic chemotherapy. And now Robert had to start his IV. He murmured something to the nurse and nodded to the mother who was trying to sleep while she wept in a makeshift bed in the corner of the small room. Robert looked down at the agitated and fearful child. An old veteran at six, he knew what was coming.

Over the past two years, little Joseph Stinson had probably had a thousand needle sticks. Blood for this study, blood for that study, new drugs for this, new chemotherapy for that. And the bone marrows, the bone marrows were absolute nightmares, and he had been subjected to a lot of those too. So everytime he saw one of these young men in white come in the night, he knew what it was for. Another IV gone bad. Time for yet more pain.

Joseph's six-year-old mind understood a great deal about the practice of medicine. He understood fever, chills, and fatigue. He understood the pain, the pain of leukemia and the pain of the bone marrow probe, and the constant needle sticks. He understood infection and antibiotics. Bleeding and blood transfusions were part of his knowledge as well. His "cure" statistic might look good for the FCI, but to him it had been two years of complete, unrelenting hell, an eternal parade of hair loss, nausea and vomiting, and the pain of needles, doctors, nurses, and students gaping at him. And now another young doctor with a needle.

Robert felt around the young boy's arm, but there were no sites left. Every vein was bruised and hardened from his previous chemotherapy. So Robert looked down at the child's legs and feet, and again puncture sites abounded. He looked hesitantly at the nurse.

"Well, I'm going to try the scalp."

"But, Dr. Gordon, we don't use the scalp on children over the age of four." The nurse tried to suppress her abhorrence.

"I know," he responded. "But he simply doesn't have any peripheral veins, and I think I can get an IV started up on the left side of his head."

So Robert proceeded as the nurse held little Joseph's head solidly in the bed. Joseph was cooperative. He had long since given up fighting. Robert's gut wrenched with pity at what he knew he had to do. All these procedures looked cruel to the casual observer. Even the seasoned physician who had started many an IV in an awkward and painful place knew the scalp was the worst of all.

Robert took the fine, 23 gauge needle and felt for a slight bulging along the left temple. The complete lack of hair from all the "chemo" made the scalp barren and smooth. He cleaned the area with alcohol and under the bright light of the nurse's lamp, neatly inserted the needle. The dark red liquid flowed back through the plastic line, and it was clear he had entered the vein correctly and precisely on the first attempt. The needle was taped up and covered in a way that would allow Joseph to roll around in the bed and not lose the IV line. Both the nurse and Robert were expert in the wrapping process.

Joseph peered up at Robert with what looked like tired admiration. The thanks were obvious in his luminous blue eyes. "You didn't hurt me, doctor. It didn't hurt!" Joseph had had many young physicians come in, and most were not as adroit with the needle as this one. He had been braced for at least three painful attempts. And here this doctor had solved the problem with one neat stick. Oh, how he wished the parade would stop and it would always be this doctor when it was time for the needle!

Robert Gordon was a star among stars. In his five years at the FCI, he had worked day and night, caring for sick patients, forging ahead in the laboratory, and publishing paper after paper in the most respected journals. And he did it all through hard work, rather than influence. He worked independently but also in collaboration with others, and he did it in laboratories that were productive, yet not part of the central axis of the FCI drug development program. His growing reputation as both a researcher and a physician were acknowledged throughout the institute.

Robert first worked as a clinical associate, his first year solely with patients, and his second in the laboratory. In contrast to most of his associates, whose interests were sharply focused on drug development, Robert was fascinated by the immune system. By observing the effects of the drugs he saw they were often effective, slowing down the growth of tumors and sometimes stopping the cancer altogether. But he also saw that patients on chemotherapy, like little Joseph, nearly always developed severe, and sometimes lethal, side effects. Drugs seemed a rather limited and barbaric tool for cancer treatment.

On the other hand, the field of immunology offered almost incomprehensible power. Robert was particularly enthralled with the incredible selectivity of the immune system. Here you had a highly organized collection of cells and antibodies that could distinguish between 20 different types of adenovirus causing the common cold, between six different types of pneumococcus, and he thought, between hundreds and perhaps thousands of different types of cancer. Here was a system that had a level of diversity and specificity which was, at least potentially, a match for cancer. And unlike drugs, which were very simple tools, really just toxic chemicals designed to kill cancer cells along with whatever healthy cells lay in the way, immunological approaches offered the possibility of a highly selective attack on the cancer cell - with less damage, if any, to normal tissues.

Yet all was not well in the field of immunotherapy.

Robert Gordon wasn't the first man of medicine to revere the mysterious workings of the immune system and envision how it might be bolstered or rerouted to squelch cancer. Paul Ehrlich had searched for antibodies as "magic bullets" to cure cancer before 1900 and, at the turn of the century, a New York physician, William Coley, began documenting the apparently miraculous "spontaneous" cancer recoveries that he and others had noted from time to time following a bout of bacterial infection. And so a man with an inoperable cancer in the neck completely recovered following a near-fatal skin infection. Another with a resistant facial sarcoma recovered following a strep throat. A young woman with advanced melanoma was alive ten years after complete disappearance of her cancer during an episode of viral hepatitis. She turns yellow and the black cancer disappears. Could something in the bacteria or viruses trigger a component of the immune system that trampled the cancer along with the infection?

As the cases mounted, Coley began fooling with concoctions of bacterial extracts, even intentionally infecting some cancer patients with what would become known as "Coley's toxins". Sometimes it worked, mostly it didn't, in the hands of Coley and others. No one understood how it worked, but Coley, and later his daughter, suspected that something in the bacterial brews was indeed lending a hand to the patients' immune systems. In a sense, through Coley's controversial toxins, immunotherapy was born.

But it was to remain controversial.

Not much success followed Coley's death in 1936. The FDA's Kefauver Act of 1962, dubbed Coley's toxins as drugs, sounded a death knell for the embryonic field. The sheer bureaucratic effort now required to purify and test bacterial extracts for immune stimulation proved too much for most investigators. In 1965, when Coley's toxins appeared on an American Cancer Society list of unproven treatments, it fell into even stronger disfavor. It seemed that harnessing the immune system to fight cancer was destined to remain as historical tidbits and anecdotes, rather than being used in the large-scale, controlled trials through university and government "thought leaders", that are behind solid, accepted science.

But the occasional miracle cures continued.

Everson and Cole compiled an interesting book on the "spontaneous regression of cancer". They documented, in a precise and scientific way, that incurable cancers very rarely regress without specific treatment. Sometimes, in line with Coley's clinical observations, an infection seemed to have played a role. Mostly, no obvious reason was found. The authors speculated that immune activation was involved and demonstrated that these regressions were most common in kidney cancer and melanoma.

In the 1960s, interest in the immune system resurfaced. Researchers transplanted miniscule bits of tumors into laboratory animals, and attempted to shrink them with various immune system extracts. But the experiments had a built-in catch - the implanted tumors (not at all a model of how a human develops cancer) consisted of a mere million cells. Everyone knew that the smallest detectable human tumor had at least 100 million cells. So what good was the immunotherapy, if it couldn't be applied soon enough?

Yet hundreds of studies were conducted, mostly on laboratory animals, some on humans. Some used bacterial preparations not much different from Coley's toxins. Tumor cells were used as vaccines. The first studies were done on the blood cancers, then on cancers of the lung, breast, colon and skin. And while most of these studies yielded marginal or frankly negative results, a very few gave positive observations. As a result, mainstream science believed immunotherapy for human cancer just didn't work. At least not in advanced cancer, which was the main problem for patients and oncologists.

Rather than accepting the dogma on the negative studies, Robert was intrigued by those few positive studies. If the idea of immunotherapy was truly off base, then it should never work, he reasoned. So Robert decided to look a little more closely at the data and experimental protocols than most of his colleagues. And, like Coley, he saw something that others missed.

Maybe it wasn't the immune system that had the problem; perhaps design of the experiments was the problem. The immune system's twin calling card was its diversity and specificity, Robert mused. So any experiment would have to use very pure extracts and reagents. But how could that be accomplished when an organism's response to imagim - whether by infection or theoretically by a cancer - was to produce a smorgasbord of biochemicals? Take antibodies. Different cells would zero in on different portions of the offending substances, like the eight blind men feeling different parts of an elephant; each expressing a different view of the beast. Each cell would then churn out its own type of antibody, so that the overall result was an organism filled with a hopelessly inseparable mixture of antibody types. How could a researcher obtain a pure preparation, so that one antibody type could be tested at a time? It simply couldn't be done. The body made these biological substances in such minute amounts that extracting enough from donors was simply not feasible.

And the problem wasn't limited to antibodies - there were other immune system substances, like the interferons and interleukins, that were in short supply. Maybe all that was needed was a way to isolate immune system components, then to make workable amounts of them. Maybe amplification in the laboratory was the key, he thought. But that was a tall technological order.

Robert also realized that more needed to be learned about the basic biology of the cancer cell. Maybe it wasn't quite as different from normal cells as many scientists thought. So while researchers sought the elusive virus causing cancer, maybe they should instead be looking for cell surface characteristics clustered perhaps uniquely on the renegade cells, but also found on some normal cells at much lower densities. Clearly, the subtleties of cell biology in general and immunology in particular had to be worked out before anyone could expect to harness their inherent properties.

But Robert recognized a less esoteric gap. By reading broadly in the immunology journals, he realized that exciting things were indeed happening in the laboratory. But these revelations generated publications, not clinical results. Scientific reputations were being built on immunology, but patients were not being helped. In fact, by 1970, immunotherapy had become a dirty word, particularly at the chemotherapy-happy FCI. Robert remained intrigued by immunotherapy, but he put it on a temporary back burner, while he turned his attention to the star of the 1970s, chemotherapy.

But in 1973, his appetite for immunotherapy was again whetted by a year's sabbatical in England, in a laboratory focused on the lymphocyte responses of mice and rats to injected proteins. These proteins were similar to the substances that made cancer cells different from their normal counterparts. It was amazing what progress the English were making with small laboratories, antiquated equipment and budgets that would be considered "petty cash" at the FCI. Robert spent his entire sabbatical probing the fascinating repertoires of lymphocytes, coming to agree with the Nobel laureate Professor Peter Medawer that each cancer was unique to each patient, and that one day, the power of the immune system could be brought to bear on this problem.

If Robert had chosen to take his sabbatical just two years later, he would have found himself in the laboratory of two other men who would also win the Nobel prize. And in one of those out of date, small English laboratories, they were to discover what would, ultimately, make all of Robert's dreams come true.

January 1975

Well, it was decision time. Robert and Mary Margaret sat across from friends at "their" corner table in their favorite Washington Italian restaurant. Carol was a nurse on the Oncology floor at the Clinical Center, and Bill was a clinical scientist, like Robert. Bill's interest was in growth and maturation factors, another area that wasn't "popular" at the FCI. However, he had plugged ahead to make a name for himself and felt that growth and maturation factors would be important in cancer treatment one day. Mary Margaret and Carol were listening intently as Robert and Bill debated vigorously.

"I don't care what kind of job you were offered at the university. There is simply no place with greater opportunity to do science than the FCI," Bill stated defiantly. "Sure, there's lots of politics, difficulties, but you'll find that at a university too. And here we have so many resources. No grants to write, no tenure review, no real difficulty with supplies or personnel to carry out your experiments. You can't say that about the university."

"True," responded Robert, "but I'm bothered by a certain lack of intellectual freedom here. I've always had the feeling that support can be cut off in one day if my laboratory chief were to leave or if the clinical chief position changed hands. Only those people working in chemotherapy development look secure. All the rest of us working on the outskirts appear to be on very shaky ground."

"Well, you're right, I suppose," conceded Bill. "But is it really different elsewhere? The FCI provides most of the cancer research money in this country anyway, and the only difference is that if you take the money at a university, you simply have to wait 12 months longer to get it. The same problems come up. You know that grant committees are set up to favorably review drug development research, and just like here in Washington, you're going to have difficulty in Atlanta."

"I know, but somehow the university should have more flexibility. I think I can recruit funds from philanthropic donors, from private corporations, from individuals who might want to support my research efforts. If this can be done, I may develop more flexible sources of support for my laboratories and clinical work outside government. That will give me the opportunity to carry out some of the experiments that I've not been able to do inside this system," Robert responded.

"I just don't know. You're talking about a position as head of medical oncology at Mallory University. I bet you'll get bogged down in committee assignments, patient care responsibilities, and administrative details that you can't even imagine now. That fund-raising sounds great, but it may take more time than writing grants. I spoke to Bruno Fisher, head of oncology at Downstate for five years now. His gripe was constant interference by the dean and administrative people in carrying out his programs in the university. My guess is you'll be trading one set of problems for another."

Robert had given the matter a great deal of thought, and he suspected Bill was right. No matter where you went, there was still an enormous effect of the "system" on cancer research and treatment. The university cancer centers were modeled after, and often attempted to function as mini-FCIs. Fortunately, Mallory had not successfully developed a federal cancer center; its efforts were more in the private sector. As a small, southern university, it had long depended upon philanthropic wealth for many of its research programs. In fact, the new clinic and laboratory that Robert was to occupy, should he accept the offer, would be built with funds from the Coke Foundation, all Coca-cola money. Drink a Coke and cure cancer, he mused.

And then there was the issue of location. Robert realized how badly Mary Margaret wanted to move back south, realized it even more as he listened to the two women now chatter back and forth about houses, children, schools. The East Coast scene had been as awful for her, a constant bickering among the wives of the physicians and scientists on who was better than who. "My husband did this, my husband won that, my husband gave a lecture to so-and-so," Mary Margaret would sarcastically repeat before she had finally taken all the Eastern back-stabbing and gossip she could tolerate. She had given up attending the social events in which women were expected to live fully through their husbands. So the Gordons had a very limited social life, and they looked forward to these Friday night Italian dinners with the Andersons, who also had that Midwestern forthrightness with which they had grown up.

Carol sympathized with her lonely friend. "I think that you and Robert should go to Atlanta immediately. I've been a nurse here for ten years. The process chews up good people. Clinical associates come here with fire in their bellies and great thoughts in their minds, hoping to change the world and do cancer research for patients. They often go away thinking in terms of how much money they can make, or how to get into this research system or that, and they become focused on exploiting the system, rather than helping people. Robert, you have an unusual sense of direction, and a real commitment to help patients. You can apply your talents best, I think, in a university environment. If you stay here, the system will eat away at you, year after year. Think about it."

"Hey, wait a minute Carol. Are you saying that I'm evolving into an Eastern bad guy? Should we leave too?" Bill asked, a little hurt and angry.

"Come on Bill, you know your work is primarily in the laboratory, and you have sequestered yourself away into your own little world. You'll continue to work and be productive by avoiding the issue."

"What do you mean?"

"I think your position and Robert's are very different. Robert thinks pragmatically, and wants to adjust and fix the system. You think specifically and want to do experiments to publish. What you can ignore, may just destroy Robert."

Carol didn't realize just how on the mark she was, Robert thought as he finished up his spaghetti. He had to face facts. With the current Musso/Lizzard axis of chemotherapy development firmly in place, there'd have to be a major breakthrough in immunology for it to receive any attention at all here. And it would have to come soon. Although Robert's contributions in the all-popular area of drug development were not insignificant - including new approaches for treating fibrohistiocytic sarcoma and small cell lung cancer - he wanted to do so much more. And he was beginning to see that he'd never be able to do it at the FCI.

It was time to move on.

The Cancer Center at Mallory University was about to get underway. The Dean and search committee members wanted Robert Gordon, and they wanted him badly.

What they had, so far, was a team of laboratory scientists and a hospital full of patients, but no connection between the two. And if there was one thing that Robert Gordon was noted for, it was his exceptional ability to bring new findings from the laboratory to the clinic, and do so expeditiously. Both his publishing record and his reputation with patients were impeccable.

The only item that caused the dean some concern was Gordon's growing reputation as a renegade, someone who wanted to change an imperfect system rather than sit back and accept it. The man may be brilliant and on target in his criticism of the cancer research system, the dean thought, but he wasn't known for his patience or his diplomacy.

But the dean saw a little bit of himself in Robert, and respected him for it. He had been patient enough to stay around as dean, but impatient to get new programs up and running. He felt that Robert would mature in the job and become the kind of leader who could make things happen without getting into battle after battle with his colleagues. So he had offered a quarter of a million dollars of Coke Foundation money to set up Robert's laboratory and to hire his initial team of scientists and technicians. In addition, he committed medical school resources to the building of the Oncology/Hematology Clinic and gave Robert rather broad control over the area of cancer treatment at Mallory. Robert would work under "Bingo" Jones, chairman of the department of medicine and elder statesman at Mallory. In spite of his nickname, "Bingo" Jones was a man who moved slowly and conservatively on everything. The interaction between the staid Dr. Jones and the revolutionary young Gordon would be interesting indeed.

July 1975

Robert Gordon did indeed go to Mallory with his wife and four children. And they thrived. Mary Margaret found a beautiful home in a wooded area near the hospital, and Robert's salary could finally allow them to live in more comfort. They found a new Italian restaurant, and now could afford to order more than the standard spaghetti dish. They didn't miss the cramped apartments and snobbery of Washington. It was great to be home in the South.

Everyone here was helpful and friendly. The bank opened their account with smiles and without pages and pages of paperwork. Mallory made them an interest-free loan for the house, and they moved in in the midst of a summer heat wave, just as they had moved into the cramped efficiency in Washington five years earlier. And within days, Mary Margaret became active in a circle of friends who supported university activities and shared a common southern heritage. She was happy.

Robert was happy too, and busy. He built a new clinic, and then began staffing the outlying clinics in the system. Next, he used the resources provided by the dean to establish a small immunology laboratory and to hire a biochemist and an immunologist. He was thrilled to be able to pursue his experiments in B cell activation and T cell killing.

Like any young investigator, much of Robert's time was spent in writing FIH grant proposals, and to his frustration, he was accumulating quite a pile of "pink sheets", the standard rejection forms. He could almost predict what they would say. "Good science and good work, but too avant-garde, too preliminary, can't be done, needs more information. Approved without funding." It was bizarre, this category of grant review; not rejected; not approved and funded; but a third category approved without funding. It was a good out for the system.

Robert was up against the famous peer review system, supposedly a system whereby each researcher's grant was objectively considered by experts in the field, in reality a stack-the-deck "old boy" system in which the design of a committee often determined who did and who didn't get funding. For example, if a committee member was asked to review a project which he already had in mind, the result was obvious. A simple "approved not funded" decision gave the reviewer time to tune up his own research grant application for the next cycle. It wasn't at all rare for the senior investigators, the ones who lead and staffed the committees, to deliberately keep another's research program floundering for years for lack of funds. So Robert accumulated his pink sheets with mounting despair.

But he plugged on. His grants in antibody toxin conjugates were not funded, but he managed to secure some FCI contract money by initiating a research project to link drugs to antibodies, and in this way could continue his work in immunology. As long as the word "drug" was in there, it would pass peer review. And Robert continued to have success in the chemotherapeutic treatment of sarcomas and lung cancer, and achieved national recognition in setting up the Mallory Cancer Treatment Center as a model referral system for the southeast region. He established the fellowship training program and joined the Southeastern Oncology Clinical Group (SOCG) with six FCI-trained oncologists that he brought on board.

But soon the lack of funds began to slow Robert's research endeavors. It seemed that every time they had a lead, they ran short of cash. The private money from the Coke Foundation was available in small quantities, and Robert could see that they would never get sufficient resources to make a truly serious effort in cancer treatment. Each grant or contract averaged $50,000 to $100,000. Any one investigator would need 10 or 15 of these grants to make a major effort in developing new treatments using biological approaches.

Only those firmly in the FCI pipeline could succeed, those investigators whose programs sucked in millions each year, yet hadn't been carefully reviewed in a decade. He also noted that like his Vietnam era clinical associate colleagues at the FCI, these well-funded programs tended to cluster on the two coasts. It was becoming increasingly difficult to see how his small group at Mallory was ever going to break into the pipeline, particularly since his research was not directly drug-oriented.

November 1975

It was Sam Luria's physician, Dr. Randall, who had suggested that his patient see Dr. Gordon, the new head of oncology at Mallory. And now, on the day of his discharge, Sam anxiously anticipated his first meeting with the much talked-about new physician.

He hoped it wouldn't be the kind of encounter he'd had all too frequently, the doctor in the long white coat walking in, looking the patient over at some distance, making a few pronouncements to his entourage, then leaving, without so much as touching or a greeting to the patient, the subject of the intense looks and scribblings. Such "attending physicians" were a royal pain in the ass as far as Sam was concerned. They had absolutely no interest in the patient, the "case", as they so often put it. They simply wanted to look good on rounds.

With a brief knock, Dr. Gordon entered the room. There was no entourage. He came right over to the bedside and shook Sam's hand firmly.

"Well, how are you feeling today, Mr. Luria?" he asked.

"Doctor, my back is better. I think the pain medication has helped. I understand that you are to discuss treatment options with me."

"Yes, I'd like to get you started on Alkeran and Prednisone. As you may have understood, these two drugs are fairly effective in the treatment of myeloma. Alkeran is a drug that kills the myeloma cells to some extent, and Prednisone may be active in that regard, or as supportive treatment during the Alkeran chemotherapy. We don't know the precise mechanism of action of this drug combination, but we do know that it is often effective in treating patients like yourself."

Sam immediately felt the impact of that last sentence. Dr. Gordon was speaking of treating him as a patient, not treating the disease. So many of the students, interns and residents who had been around were focused on the disease. Sam often felt like he was a multiple myeloma lying in a bed. He wondered what a breast cancer might look like. Instead, this doctor was talking about him as a patient, a person, with myeloma. It was a great, if subtle, difference.

"Well, I'm ready to take my medicine, doctor, but I have several questions. What will happen to my stem cell compartment? How long will the Alkeran work? What effect will it have on my platelets? Will my cells become resistant to these drugs? Just how toxic are they? How long can I take Alkeran? Is it true that the drug causes other kinds of cancer when taken for a long period of time?"

"Hold it, hold it," Dr. Gordon interrupted. "I can't answer all of those questions at once. Where have you picked up all of this information?" He was clearly surprised at the depth of his new patient's knowledge.

"Well, I've been down in the medical library, and I've also had the opportunity to talk to some of my friends, thanks to the phone here." He looked rather lovingly at the phone next to his bed. "Being in the restaurant business for so long, Doc, I've got a lot of friends in medical circles who come to me for regular doses of souvlaki. So I've been picking their brains, you might say."

"Indeed you have."

"I'm really interested in learning more about the immune system, which I understand is your specialty," Sam continued, moving around a little more as he got into his favorite subject. "Why can't we make an antibody to kill my myeloma cells and avoid all these toxic drugs? Maybe I should run off to the Bahamas, I understand their treatments are non-toxic," Sam laughed.

"You're right there, those treatments are non-toxic, but they're also non-effective," Dr. Gordon answered, moving a little closer. "But with regard to the antibody issue, you have actually hit upon an area of intense interest for me. It does seem reasonable and logical that we should be able to make antibodies and use them in the treatment of a patient like yourself. The problem is that every time we make antibodies against cancer cells, we can't seem to make the same exact antibody twice. We inject a rabbit with cancer cells, and sometimes it will make a serum similar to an earlier preparation, but more often than not, it churns out new types of antibodies each time, or just rolls over and dies. This inability to reproduce our results is very frustrating.

"Well, doctor, is the problem conceptual, or do you simply need more hands?" Sam asked.

By this time Dr. Gordon had forgotten he was talking to a patient, and carried on as if he were conversing with another immunologist. "It's both. Certainly, if I had more technicians, we could make more antibodies, but I don't want to kid you, I think there are some pretty basic technological problems. No matter how many hands we have, we'll always have trouble making large amounts of uniform preparations of antibody by injecting rabbits. It's just too long and laborious a process, and we need more precise methods."

"Well, back to me doctor. I intend to take the Alkeran and Prednisone and come see you in the clinic in a month. I want you to think about making those antibodies. Don't you think it would be interesting to use the antibodies along with T cell stimulation and perhaps a macrophage activator? Do you think you can eventually do that for me?"

"Well, not yet. But there is the possibility of experimental protocols in the future. Let's get you started on chemotherapy, and then we can discuss the other possibilities later. In the meantime, you keep reading. I have a feeling you are going to educate me in the long run, Mr. Luria. Now, get some rest." When they parted, both men were smiling.

The new head of oncology had done more to help Sam's frame of mind than anything yet in his fight with cancer. He had treated him not only as a patient, but as a person, and not only as a person, but as a person who was his intellectual peer. He could hardly wait to get back to his WATTS line and set his personal immunotherapy plan into action.

He was certain that he and the Doc would make quite a team.

At precisely the time of the initial meeting between Sam Luria and Robert Gordon, several dozen mice in a laboratory at the Medical Research Council in England were already providing an answer to the technological roadblock Robert had described. The mice had been manipulated by a young scientist named Georges Kohler, who had come to the Medical Research Council laboratories to work with the great immunologist, Cesar Milstein, just two years after Robert Gordon, in a laboratory down the hall. Kohler too, had sought a way to make the elusive antibodies more accessible.

He had an idea. And like most scientific breakthroughs destined for the history books, Kohler's was astonishingly simple. And therein lay its beauty.

What Georges Kohler did was to enlist the aid of cancer cells, an unlikely but brilliant strategy. Specifically, what he did was to harness the never-ending cell division of the cancer cell growing in tissue culture. He took a B cell from a mouse that had been injected with an antigen, a bit of sheep blood. In response, the mouse's immune system churned out the appropriate B cells, each one a mini-factory of just one antibody type. Each antibody fits like a key, into some lock on the sheep blood cells' surfaces. The foreign blood cells, dotted with clinging antibodies, called attention to the invader and signaled other components of the immune system to come in for the kill. Soon the mouse's blood was crawling with a host of different antibodies, each able to grab onto the sheep blood cells at a different point.

But all Kohler needed was one B cell, a potential template for a single antibody type. Now the trick was to isolate it and get it to thrive outside the mouse, and conveniently coax it to pump out its product for the young investigator. B cells, however, are notoriously finicky about just where they will grow, and most die off in the tissue culture bottle. Kohler, though, had a formidable trick up his sleeve.

He managed to isolate a B cell, and before it conked out on him, fuse it with another cell, a mouse cancer cell. The cancer cells came from a mouse myeloma, a disease similar to Sam Luria's. These myeloma cells were like factories, able to produce antibodies in large quantities. And they grew like weeds in the laboratory. They usually produced lots of the wrong antibodies in the test tube and in patients like Sam. The trick was to use the factory to produce the "right" antibody. In the fall of 1975, Kohler fused B cells and myeloma cells, "fed" them, and then left them alone for awhile, to see what would grow out. He was looking for a particular marriage of cells, an artificially concocted cell that would retain the antibody-producing capabilities of an activated B cell, and the "immortality" of the cancerous myeloma cell.

And just about Christmas time, when Sam Luria and Robert Gordon were deep into their dialog about the seeming impossibility of harnessing antibodies for cancer treatment, Kohler and Milstein's mice were discovering the solution.

The sought-after fusion cell; a cross between a B cell and a myeloma cell, a veritable antibody factory that could live on in the lab forever, became known as a hybridoma, and its oh-so-valuable product, monoclonal antibodies.

They would revolutionize medicine.

CHAPTER 12

PRIZES LARGE AND SMALL

1980

They were New York's finest, and this had nothing to do with the police force.

The scene was the Waldorf Astoria, the very best ballroom, ready for the very best people. All of the scions of New York society were on hand, the men in black tie, the women trying to outdo each other with their designer evening gowns. Doormen rushed to greet each arriving limousine, ushering the couples into the cocktail party with a formal "Dr. and Mrs. Andrew Martin Seymour Hurley have arrived."

It was the annual Wilson banquet.

At the top of the enormous staircase, THE Mrs. Wendell Wilson stood regally dressed to greet her hundreds of invited guests. She was a small and exceedingly elegant woman who held her chin, and some said her nose, high. Her white hair, expensive gown, meticulous make-up were all in perfect accord. She looked down the stairs at her friends, associates, and sometime competitors arriving for her party. She had given it for 15 years as the culmination of the competition for the coveted Wilson Prize.

Winning the Wilson Prize was the dream of every researcher, an acknowledged stepping stone to the still greater Nobel Prize. It was presented each year by the slight Mrs. Wilson in memory of her husband, who had died of lung cancer, caused by his two packs a day of cigarettes, in the mid 1960s. And although she and her husband had never been very interested in cancer research until it directly affected them, she had become involved shortly after his death when a good friend and family physician had outlined the opportunity for her. Of course she knew she couldn't financially match the offering of the dynamite king, Alfred Nobel, but she revelled in the accolades surrounding her contribution. She was completely satisfied being the Avis of the Prize business.

Mrs. Wilson descended the stairs like a Queen. The jewelled guests filed past, each remark more inane than the last. "Your dress is beautiful!", "My, you look wonderful!", "The decorations are exquisite this year!" She basked in the compliments.

People often wondered how such a frail widow could have so much power. From her base in New York society, her tentacles reached out across the nation, and most particularly to that rather small town to the south, Washington, D.C. In addition to her ability to influence research with her Prize, she had, through her friends and associates, considerable political influence in the halls of Congress. Over the years, more than one piece of health legislation had been passed as a result of her lobbying efforts. By selectively pushing this Senator and that Representative, she was often able to get things done that no one else could possibly accomplish. The prestige of the Wilson Prize and, of course, her family's immense wealth and influence, had a great deal to do with her success. But others had money and connections, and didn't carry half her clout. Her secret was as much a mystery as the scientific problems she sought to unravel through her Prize.

Mrs. Wilson held court at the head table, surrounded by her various cronies, representing society, the medical profession, academia, government and industry. To her right was the current President of the Wilson Foundation, Mr. Chauncey Armstrong. His regal-sounding name came from a Duke a few generations back, and he had been a friend of Mr. Wilson. As the aristocratic gentleman rose and made his way to the podium, the audience grew still. The great moment was approaching.

"Ladies and gentlemen, it has given me supreme pleasure to have been President of the distinguished Wilson Foundation for the past year. As you well know, this banquet signifies the end of one person's term and the beginning of another's. I know you will all be interested to learn of Mrs. Wilson's selection for the incoming president, but I would first like to enjoy the final brief moments of my year by announcing the winner of the 1980 Wendell Wilson Prize in cancer research." Armstrong was a man who loved to be in the spotlight. He had a wonderful English accent, although it was said that in private he would often lapse into speech that was pure New York.

"As most of you know, the Wilson Prize has been awarded for the last 15 years, and in no less than 10 of those years, a Wilson Prize winner has subsequently become a Nobel Laureate. I think this record clearly demonstrates the great wisdom and foresight of the Wilson committee in selecting each year's winner. I have no doubt that this year's winner will continue the tradition. He is a man of great vision, a man of great accomplishment, and a man mature beyond his years. Over the last decade, he has repeatedly led science into new areas of inquiry and has been at the forefront in his field of investigation. He and Dr. George Trumpey coined this new term "oncogene", which has become well known by now to most cancer biologists. A fearsome word, a word which means a gene that causes cancer."

"While it is still unclear just what role oncogenes play in the causation of human cancer, it is clear that they exist and they are critical in some way. Tonight's Wilson Prize winner not only coined the term and described the first oncogene protein product, but he has been a leader in the field of molecular biology for more than a decade."

As Chauncey Armstrong stopped to take a drink, murmuring traveled throughout the audience. At the first use of the word "oncogene", nearly everyone there had known who the winner was. Michael Chapman. A little young, perhaps, but quite brilliant and most deserving. Dr. Chapman had started his post graduate training at Harvard, and later at the FCI under George Trumpey. He became a senior investigator and later head of the Laboratory of Molecular Biology at UCLA, where he was given sufficient resources and laboratory space to build a premiere molecular biology team during the late 1970s. A tireless worker and a man respected by all of his colleagues, both because of the quality and insight of his work and the force of his personality, Michael Chapman certainly deserved the praise he was to receive that evening.

At a prominent center table, the mood was especially cheerful. Stephen Musso and his wife and Roger Salla and his friend sat talking animatedly with some members of the Wilson family. Roger's girlfriend looked over a few tables to Dr. Chapman admiringly, almost like a teenager might gaze at a rock star, and whispered, "Dr. Chapman seems to be a very successful scientist. And so young! Do you know him?"

Roger thought he could see her begin to drool. He bent down to her, an amused smirk on his lips, "Yes, yes, I know Michael very well. He is a good scientist, a damn good one. But even with the recent grant from the John Wayne Foundation, he lacks the resources to finish to work he's begun, and he's somewhat focused, exploring many areas simultaneously rather than trying to reach a singular goal."

"But why should availability of resources be a factor in evaluating someone's worth as a scientist?" she asked.

"Resources are everything," Roger answered somewhat distractedly, as he watched the pretty people on the podium. "To be serious about molecular biology, you must have major resources."

"Like you do ..."

"As a matter of fact, yes." Sometimes Roger couldn't quite tell whether she was being naive or sarcastic. But he continued. "We have the laboratory to solve some of the big problems in molecular biology, and I think our work with viruses will ultimately prove more valuable than the current work with oncogenes," he said.

She guessed his answer was tinged a little with sour grapes, but she enjoyed egging him on. "Well, aren't oncogenes just viruses that are in the cell on a more or less permanent basis, sort of marooned viruses?"

"Yes, in a sense that's true, but with a major difference," Roger responded. They had met when he spoke in a graduate seminar where she was a student, and couldn't help sounding somewhat professorial at times, although his interest in her was not primarily intellectual. "The oncogene is really integrated, and a functional part of the genetic apparatus of a cell. Some of these may come along with us from the very beginning. On the other hand, viruses function within the cell without total integration, and most are acquired after birth. Both are important, but I think viruses will ultimately play the larger role in understanding cancer biology."

Stephen Musso had caught bits of Roger's speech, and leaned closer. "You're right on target, Roger. Michael Chapman may be a sharp cookie, but you've got the resources to whip him one day. I'm gonna see that you continue to have those resources. You will win the big Prize before him."

He continued. "In fact, I think there's a good chance you'll be on that podium next year, the winner of the 1981 Wilson Prize. Then, it will be a horse race to see who can get the Nobel Prize first. Will it be for the oncogene or the viral theory of cancer causation? If you can get that work finished we discussed on the lymphoma virus, you're a shoo-in for the Wilson Prize. And then I can reorganize George Trumpey's laboratory and give you even more resources."

"Stephen, we're very close, and I think the announcement on the lymphoma virus can be made within six weeks. I'm looking forward to being the chief of the combined laboratories we discussed." And, I'm looking forward to getting rid of that jerk Trumpey as well, he thought with real pleasure.

But he knew that as spectacular as the lymphoma announcement would be, he wouldn't receive all the glory.

Stephen would take a great deal of credit for it. Well, that would even the score for the leukemia virus fiasco. And then Roger would stun everyone with the colon cancer breakthrough. No one could snatch that one from him, or sabotage it. And it would be so much bigger!

Each year 20,000 people were diagnosed with lymphoma. But 100,000 received a verdict of colon cancer. Plus, colon cancer strikes important people in their most productive years. There was simply no question which discovery would have the greater impact. Roger meant to ride the winning horse.

He couldn't wait.

Stephen Musso set about designing the peer review committee to destroy George Trumpey with great enjoyment.

Trumpey had been around long enough. Year after year he was a thorn in Musso's side. George simply refused to check with Stephen on announcements and progress from his laboratory. He was independent. Each year Stephen would make the appropriate announcements on curing cancer with drugs, and each year George would divert the attention of the media with his work on oncogenes and viruses. George just didn't know when to shut up. He was an able spokesman and continued to divert attention from what Stephen considered to be mainstream FCI work. Plus, George's laboratory of viral oncology was huge, second only to Roger Salla's. Stephen meant to right that situation, and this committee would do the trick.

Everything was in place. The review was scheduled for next month, and Stephen had meticulously selected just those committee members who were both highly respected and highly critical of Trumpey's work. Musso was a pro at designing committees to give desired results, and he wanted to make sure that this review group came to the right conclusion. Over the years Stephen had kept careful tabs on who was jealous of George, or who resented his work for one reason or another, but who had remained, at least on the surface, friendly to him.

And so with these people constituting the committee, no one would suspect (or prove) the deck had quite literally been stacked. Peer review would all look fair and square. As always. And George would be found wanting.

Just as Stephen Musso was a pro in ferreting out personal information and then using it to further his ends, Daniel Jenkins, the head of Trumpey's committee, also was a pro. Danny's specialty was feigning friendship and then stabbing people in the back. Nicknamed "Hi-Jinx" for his practical jokes, he had a major grant from the FCI to fund his oncogene research at Duke, and a full understanding of the way Stephen Musso wanted things to turn out. And so he was well prepared to subtly lead the discussion to crucify Trumpey.

Danny didn't really have anything against George Trumpey, in fact he enjoyed the way he expertly handled the questions from the press. But Danny had a great, yet simple, need. More funding.

His $5 million FCI grant was up for renewal in the fall. Stephen, in the same sentence, had assured him that his proposal was among the best he'd seen, and he was sure that the Trumpey review would go well. To anyone else it would seem a non sequitur, but Danny read the message clearly. He knew Stephen was irritated by George's independence, and had placed his bet on Salla as the government's leading virologist. Danny also knew that Trumpey's lab sucked up a lot of FCI money. If it was dismantled, where would it go? Maybe to fund grants. And although it was never explicitly stated, never discussed and never written, it was clearly understood that a negative review on George's work would result in a positive funding action for Danny's project and an expansion of the Salla program.

Only one week to go, Stephen thought.

Roger Salla continued to work furiously night and day. With two potential cancer viruses in the works, he hadn't time for anything frivolous. Roger completed the paper on the lymphoma virus, and pushed Charlie to work harder and harder on the colon virus. He was a man obsessed, like a runner in the last 100 yards of a mile, pushing and pushing and pushing everyone to an even greater extent than usual in his laboratory.

And he was getting results. The work was going so well that even he was surprised. In fact, the first colon paper would soon be sent off to Nature. Elevating Roger's mood even higher was the fact that George's review was coming up soon, and it would likely be negative.

For nearly two decades, the two of them had fought and competed. He had done some things to hurt George, and he was certain George had done some things to hurt him. In addition to switching cultures and spiking cells with viruses, there had been the more subtle ploys. The confrontations, major and minor, at meetings; the exclusion of one another on books, papers and symposia; the telephone character assassinations; the attempts, both overt and covert, to harm one another's professional reputation.

Now he would be free of George at last, and not only that, he would gain control of his resources. A bright new lab complex in the Arlington, Virginia facility! It wasn't enough for Roger that he had more space, contracts, personnel and equipment than any single scientist in the world. He wanted still more, for he knew well that resources spelled success. Trumpey's lab would increase his capability by nearly 40 percent, putting him in a position of dominance that could never be approached by any other investigator, anywhere. Roger knew he was both a brilliant scientist and a superb strategist. Add the limitless resources, and he knew that spelled Nobel.

Michael Chapman indeed won the 1980 Wilson Prize, and the world appropriately took notice. But a simultaneous event went almost unnoticed outside the halls of the FCI and certain select and informed university investigators.

George Trumpey's laboratory failed to pass peer review.

The summary report of the site visit, put together by the respected Daniel Jenkins, read as follows:

> *"This laboratory, although highly productive over the last decade, appears to be experiencing major difficulties. Over the last two years, productivity has dropped markedly, and the dissatisfaction on the part of junior and senior scientists is apparent. On review of the science, this committee has uncovered major deficits with respect to repeating experiments and using valid controls. The general strategy and coordination of the laboratory's endeavors are not well focused. Specifically, the work on growth factors and the viral anti-oncogene induction of such factors is not competitive with similar efforts in the university sector, and should therefore not continue to have available the same level of resources. ... Thus, our recommendation is that the FCI remove selective components, as listed below, of this laboratory and place them in other areas of the Institute where they might work more productively. This will reduce the scope of the laboratory from its current level to one of approximately one-third that size. In this way, it is hoped that this group of productive scientists can become more sharply focused and even more productive in years to come."*

Jenkins had put in a lot of time and effort crafting the report. After all, his own funding depended on it. And so the beautiful language painted a positive image of action to serve the good of the Institute, of curing cancer. The committee was just trying to help George solve his problem. Of course, poor George had been unaware there even was a problem until the committee invented one. And so his time in government research was limited.

1980 had been a banner year for Roger Salla. Major discoveries in his laboratory and the complete dismantling of his only serious competition. He was now the undisputed virus king at the FCI. Now the press would follow him around for any tidbit of information.

He now had it all. And he meant to use it well.

CHAPTER 13

THE ARLINGTON BIOTHERAPY PROGRAM AND THE TEST PILOT

February 1980

President Richard M. Nixon, when he declared his War on Cancer, said that "America will beat the swords into plowshares" in the area of science in a single master stroke to conquer cancer. He decided to shift the laboratories for biological warfare in Arlington, Virginia, to a world class cancer research center. Indeed, huge expenditures were allocated, and the FCI Arlington Cancer Research Center (ACRC) was born.

It was originally envisioned as a contract research site --- companies would compete for government contracts to manage and run the research center -- a way to expand government programs without actually adding government employees; a neat way around personnel ceilings and hiring freezes. The Arlington facility had two missions -- to provide a setting for basic research in cancer biology, and also to provide cells, viruses and biochemicals needed by FCI investigators. But to many on the Washington campus, ACRC center was viewed as a competitor, a threat rather than a supply house.

The small and select FCI Executive Committee had gathered in Stephen Musso's office. Stephen reigned supreme at the head of the shiny conference table.

"So, what I envision is a small pilot program in Arlington working on these biological substances. I've got that goddamn Mrs. Wilson on my neck calling Congressmen every third day about interferon. I've got to do something about it. As all of you well know, our chemotherapy program is much more likely to come up with more effective cancer treatment than this biological crap. I don't want to siphon off significant funds for the program. On the other hand, like a stockbroker, I think we ought to hedge our bets a bit and go ahead and create a biologicals program in case we're wrong."

The others in the room looked at each other a bit apprehensively. "What exactly do you mean, Stephen?" ventured Stanley Lizzard.

"Well, we must protect our image. It seems to me that the best of both worlds would be to institute a small ACRC program and let it operate for a few years. We need a director who is aggressive and highly capable, yet expendable. We can watch the program for 2 or 3 years, and if it's clear that biologicals are not going to become a fourth method of cancer treatment, we can simply cut the program, relocate the best people, and let the director take the rap.

"And if it works? What happens then?" asked Roger Salla.

"No sweat. Should the biological area expand and Mrs. Wilson's damned interferon or other biological substances begin to show interesting results in cancer treatment, we can take credit for having begun this innovative program at an early stage. I'm sure the director won't mind sharing his accomplishments with all of you who have provided such a prophetic opportunity."

It was classic Stephen Musso. They had all seen the strategy before. Put in a program to fill a political need, and get rid of it when the need evaporated. And the secret to success was always that excellent but expendable director. To everyone at the table, it made sense. All of them expected biologicals to become important in 5 or 10 years. But in the meantime, a not-too-large program would fill the bill, shutting up Mrs. Wilson and her friends, but keeping the FCI online with Congress should this "fourth modality" take off earlier than anticipated.

Roger was the first to mention what was obviously on everyone's mind. "Stephen, the Arlington facility's large fermentation plant supplies my researchers with viruses and cells. I want to be certain that this new program will not interrupt the flow of those essential materials to my laboratory."

Stanley seconded Roger's request, describing the drug fermentation program there.

"You both have my assurance on that," Stephen responded. "I imagine that the new director will be interested in using some of the fermentation capacity, since growing cells is a major component of making interferon and the like. However, we'll be sure that the capacity you are currently using remains within your domain.

"I have a large laboratory investigating drug resistance at Arlington," piped up Stanley Lizzard. "I surely don't want to see a negative impact by this development."

"Stanley, I want to reassure you completely on your programs at ACRC. In fact, it is my intention to put the biologicals program within your division. Since the primary focus of this program will be in developing biological substances for systemic cancer treatment, I want to be sure that it is integrated into your chemotherapy drug development program and under your direct control. There will be no negative impact on your drug resistance and fermentation programs. You'll have complete control over the development of biotherapy as well."

Stanley sat back, satisfied and somewhat smug. He didn't have much confidence in this biological business. In fact, he thought interferon was a bunch of baloney. He had looked into this "immunotherapy." A lot of animal models and papers in the literature, but no real success in patients. And these new antibodies, monoclonal antibodies, more biological hogwash. It would be easy to swallow up the dinky little program into his own.

Sam Fish went to the board. He outlined the ACRC programs. But he too had concerns and after stifled yawns attesting to a somewhat tedious presentation, he brought up a point that had been bothering him. He thought it would make a good example for Stephen and prevent future problems. "Stephen, before we worry about the future of the Arlington facility, we should clear up an existing problem there."

"Yes? What is that?"

"As you know, Jim Banner has been the director of the Biolab contract program. Since he is not a government employee, he has been a real loose cannon. He talks to every newspaper reporter who snoops around, and continues to pursue his own ends in terms of developing an ACRC power base. He's not a good team player and clearly, not one of us! He doesn't respond when we ask him to quiet down or to change a particular line of investigation. He tends to support his people very well and get them riled up in controversies that set up two sides -- Arlington vs. the FCI. I'm very concerned that he will have a damaging effect on us in the long term."

"Sam, I agree with you and I'm glad you brought it up. No action is needed today, but it's certainly on my agenda. It is a good example of just what we should be alert of. All of us ought to be looking into methods by which the ACRC can proceed quietly and well under our control. I don't need to tell you what a disaster it would be if a major accomplishment was to come out of Arlington. Of the several hundred million dollars spent on our own internal programs yearly, more than 90% stays right here in Washington. Expenditure must match accomplishment. If Congress was to think that a small amount of money spend in Arlington could result in major findings in cancer research, they would question why we're spending so damn much here without marvelous results. Banner must be watched; ACRC must remain under our control. I imagine this year will finish his tenure, and at the next review, we can restructure the contract and establish control through someone from this committee." Stephen set his gaze on Sam Fish. Another commitment had been made. Sam sat, pleased with himself.

Now Stanley stood up to cover one final issue. "As most of you know, there has been an outside committee at work helping to establish an FCI biologics program. Although most of their recommendations are benign and should cause us no difficulty -- that is, they can be implemented with minimal negative impact on our drug development programs -- there is one area of real concern."

"I think I know what you mean but go ahead," Stephen said.

"Have any of you seen the cost calculations on producing interferon?" Stantley continued. "They're astronomical. Estimates vary from $100 million to nearly a billion, for phases I, II and III clinical trials. That'll break us. Now, with Mrs. Wilson's help, we can get about $10 million from Congress for interferon trials to lessen their negative impact on drug development. It is clear to me that whomever is put at the helm of biologicals is going to push hard and we need to insure now that it's kept under control. Do we really want to dump several hundred million dollars into this stuff over the next three or four years?"

The debate that broke out lead naturally to a consideration of genetic enginnering, which would provide a far cheaper and cleaner source of interferon. All looked to Sam Fish, whose background was in microbial genetics. "How about it, Sam, what are the chances of engineering some bug to pump out interferon for us? It would certainly beat squeezing it from blood banks at $10,000 a shot," Stanley said.

"Well, it would be my guess that genetically engineered alpha interferon won't be available for another five years. I'd say 1984 at the earliest. So the problem outlined by Stanley is very real. We've got to put a cap on the blood bank source, until the gene can be cloned and bacteria coaxed to churn it out. Then we can transfer the costs to pharmaceutical companies," he concluded.

"Interferon may not be the only thing we have to consider. What about these monoclonal antibodies? Magic bullets, I think the press is calling them," piped up Allen Greenspan. Allen, head of cancer epidemiology, was a slight, jittery man, resembling Woody Allen. Because most of the people on the executive committee were treatment-oriented, Allen's opinions were rarely sought. However, he had a tendency to break in with interesting little questions, from a fresh perspective.

Everyone looked around the table to see who would lead with a response. Stephen finally did so himself.

"There is no questions that monoclonal antibodies represent an interesting technology. They may help with selectively delivering drugs to the cancer cell. However, as best as I can determine, these techniques of making antibody are still primitive, and unlikely to yield substances ready for the clinic within the next five years. In addition, they are derived from mice, and I just can't see mouse proteins as a major therapeutic substance in the long term. Sure, I've heard inklings of early success in fashioning human monoclonals, but they're nowhere near ready yet. So I don't think these "magic bullets" -- what an awful term -- will require significant resources much before 1988. But thanks for your input, Allen."

Everybody around the table nodded in agreement. "Injecting monoclonals from mice into humans is absolutely absurd," Stanley snickered. "It'll never work. Long before monoclonals are going into patients, we'll have better and better drugs available -- that is, if we keep the resources in the right places."

But little Dr. Greenspan had his doubts, although he was too timid to voice them. He'd been doing some reading. Monoclonal antibodies from mice just might work, and even if they didn't, it was only a matter of time until human versions were on the scene. The great Dr. Lizzard certainly misjudged this one, he thought. Monoclonals are going to be big news in cancer biology, and long before 1988.

Stephen stood and stretched. "Well, I guess we are all in agreement. We will make an official announcement of the biologics program and we'll locate it at ACRC. Now, I want to propose a name for it." He turned and walked slowly to the blackboard, like a famous artist about to unveil a masterpiece. He wrote in enormous letters 'FCI Biotherapy Program'.

"I want to use this word, biotherapy, because it is a logical extension of the existing three modalities in cancer treatment -- surgical therapy, radiotherapy and chemotherapy. Now, maybe biotherapy will turn out to be just so much horse manure, like immunotherapy, but let's go ahead and capture the word for the program so we will have invented it, if there's anything to it. We'll hire a director who is aggressive and productive and let him develop this program. And if it's successful, and he knows how to play the game, I'll make it possible for him to join our group to go on to bigger and better things. If he is not one of us or it is not successful, he will be expendable. In either case, we win."

Sam Fish looked up over his prinze nez glasses and asked the big question, "Stephen, do you have someone in mind to be director?" For everyone knew that he did.

"Yes, I do. I have several individuals in mind but one in particular. He is a man who I almost hired years ago. He elected instead to go to Mallory to start a new medical oncology program. He has been there about five years now and has accomplished a great deal. Given his background in immunology and his accomplishments in cancer chemotherapy, I think he may be the ideal man for this job."

This description caused the color to drain from Stanley Lizzard's face. "Stephen, surely you don't mean Robert Gordon, do you?"

"Yes, that's exactly who I mean."

"But wouldn't that cause more potential problems for Arlington?"

"What do you mean?"

"Well, like Banner, Gordon is a fellow who tends to speak his mind and get involved in controversies. He also is a very direct individual, not hesitating to speak out on issues. You may remember that during his previous tenure at the FCI, we were unable to manipulate some things with which he was involved because he simply wouldn't cooperate. Don't you think we might run into the same difficultly again?"

"Yes, and that's precisely why I want him," said Stephen. Of course he had it all worked out. "I think Robert Gordon is likely to be the same aggressive and productive person he has been for the last ten years and as such, he is likely to cause us difficulty. But he'll get the program up and going faster than anyone else could and will put himself in a position to become expendable after bringing success to it. On top of that, Stanley, he will be directly under your supervision, so I'm sure you will be able to take care of any problems that might arise from Dr. Gordon being one of your associate directors.

But Stanley didn't share Stephen's cool confidence. There was something about Gordon that had always bugged him. He wasn't at all sure he wanted him around, supervised or not.

CHAPTER 14

THE DECISION

Fall 1980

Robert Gordon continued his "rog", churning up a steep hill in the rolling woods that surrounded Mallory University. Yes, rog. His pace these days was around 7-8 minutes a mile, up from the sub 7-minutes he could manage with ease in his younger days, but not quite as bad as the 9 and 10 minute milers clad in their fancy outfits that he, in his old shorts and T-shirt, could still pass. So he was no longer a runner, but certainly he was not a jogger.

As was usually the case, his mind was churning in tempo with his legs. There must be something to his theory that the pounding of the feet releases endorphins in the brain, elevating the mood and clearing the mind. It certainly worked for him -- and was quite a bit more healthy than the cigarettes and alcohol that many of his colleagues turned to for stress relief. And today he really needed this five mile run, for once again, it was decision time.

His last big decision was in 1975, when he weighed carefully the choice of whether to join Stephen Musso as head of immunological monitoring, or whether to come to Mallory as director of oncology. Musso had been most convincing, promising him moderate responsibilities in the short term, and a rather vague assurance of expanded resources in the long term.

But Robert wasn't happy with the Musso method of uncertain futures, and had pressed him for a firmer commitment. Specifically, he'd needed at the very least two Ph.D. immunologists and a biochemist or two, along with 4 or 5 technicians to make a serious effort for the FCI in this new and very promising area. Stephen, who had expected Robert to jump at the offer, was a little put off by his queries. But Robert persistently pointed out that the new position would provide basically the same resources as his present position in the immunology branch -- the appointment would be little more than a change in name. Not giving Musso a chance to respond, a faux pas, Robert had gone on to mention the Mallory offer, and his plans to expand the program there beyond what he currently had at the FCI.

Slowly for emphasis, Stephen reiterated his original offer, and that was that. Accept or not. Robert was in a quandary. On the one hand, he knew that Stephen indeed had the resources to develop a first-rate immunology program aimed at cancer treatment. But on the other, Robert questioned Stephen's professional interest in biologicals -- wouldn't such support threaten his commitment to drug development?

Robert also recalled the 1975 atmosphere at the FCI, in which the other section chiefs behaved more like henchmen than scientists. Wasn't that one of the reasons he had left the first time? If Stephen asked them to clean the bathrooms they'd probably do it without a whimper of protest. And then there was that slimy Stanley Lizzard! Robert couldn't quite place what bothered him so much about the man. Perhaps it was the way he looked at him, maintaining eye contact just a little too long. Whatever, the more he had thought about it, the less attractive Musso's offer had seemed.

As Robert rounded the corner near the natural science building and started down the long flat stretch near the Law School, he reflected on his five years in Atlanta. Indeed, he'd had more freedom. But he had to be fair, the university could be stifling too. The dean wanted this, the Bingo wanted that, and the basic science chiefs wanted something entirely different. In every case, to garner new resources, whether it be dollars, laboratory space, or administrative support, the game was the same -- cajole your peers, convince the higher-ups, and finally get the almighty dean's approval. Was it really any different from the red tape at the FCI?

Robert thought he had been effective, his driving enthusiasm reaching out in many directions. The new hospital was completed, medical oncology services had been initiated at Memorial Hospital and the VA, and expansion of services to outlying clinics was going well. He was particularly proud of the new oncology ward, with isolation rooms for the complicated bone marrow transplants and a new orientation program for the nursing staff that was more focused on patient needs. Of course, no matter what he did, someone, somewhere was unhappy.

His research efforts were going well too. His immunologist and the biochemist, four technicians, had private support from the Coke Foundation and substantial FCI contract support. He continued his work in analyzing lymphocyte responses in cancer patients, and had stacked up an impressive publication record -- ten papers in the past year. Four were in prestigious immunology journals, another four in medical oncology journals, and two in more general scientific publications.

Despite his success in the clinic and in the laboratory, Robert remained frustrated. He felt that subtle roadblocks were being laid in place to thwart progress, particularly in the person of David Dennison, associate chairman of pathology and an expert in colon cancer. Both were vying for the position of director of the new Mallory Cancer Center. What Robert had going for him was the undeniable fact that he had singlehandedly established virtually all of the cancer treatment capability at Mallory. But what Dr. Dennison had going for him was his considerable behind-the-back influence. He was part of Mallory's "old boy" network, great pals with the dean and the basic science chairmen. More worrisome, he was married to Sarah Beth Ingram, niece of the President of Mallory. The man was, in fact, a very gifted pathologist, but he had contributed virtually nothing to Mallory's recent development as a cancer treatment center. In addition, the clinical department chairmen didn't look too kindly on the effervescent Dr. Gordon -- in fact, Robert suspected that many of them resented the resources allocated to him over the past five years. They certainly would not support his appointment as director of a new cancer center. And good old David, he was feeding those "concerns".

Robert started down the long downhill stretch towards his office, picking up speed. Towards the end of his runs he liked to imagine that he was back in high school, where he was a miler of some talent. He'd stopped running after winning the mile Tri-County regionals and placing second in the state finals, but had picked it up again 8 years ago, when he noticed that his middle was growing a bit too pudgy. He was still quite a competitor, and had done well in the various 10-K races around the Atlanta area. He felt a burst of exhiliration as he pounded down the hill into the hospital parking lot, visualizing a strong finish in this year's Peachtree Classic.

He leaned back on a red Corvette for a few minutes, closing his eyes and letting the sun dry the sweat from his face, his pounding heart and rapid breathing fading into normalcy. He studied a passing co-ed for a few minutes, then came to a decision.

He would return to the FCI.

The offer had come as quite a surprise. On the previous Monday, Robert had been revising a paper in his office, occasionally glancing out the window at the attractive nursing students leaving the adjacent nurses' dormitory, when his secretary buzzed on the intercom. "Dr. Gordon, you have a call from Dr. Musso."

Except for passing greetings at ASCO, it had been five years since he'd last spoken to Stephen. He picked up the beige phone to the left of his desk with much curiosity. "Yes, this is Dr. Gordon."

"Just a moment, please," breathed the secretary.

After a brief pause, Robert heard the voice of his old boss. "Robert! How is everything in the deep South?"

"Fine, things are going well in Atlanta. How's everything in government, Stephen?"

"Things are going reasonably well, you know, the usual inquiries and investigations, but the best of science as well. Our new drug studies and virus work are going very well." After some further "war stories", Stephen came right to the point.

"As you may have heard, we are contemplating a program to investigate biologicals in cancer treatment. In fact, a blue-ribbon panel has been actively addressing the question for the past eight months. Their conclusions have just been handed to me, and I concur. The FCI needs a dedicated program to look into these biologicals and to see what might be useful for the future."

"Stephen, didn't we go through this five years ago?"

"Wait a minute. This program is entirely different, and I am willing to totally commit myself to its launching."

"That's wonderful news! How can I help?"

"I hope you will do more than just help. The program will need the direction of someone young and aggressive who will get the job done in spite of our bureaucracy and red tape." He paused for dramatic effect, pure Musso. "And I'd like to have you come run this program for me."

Robert paused. The call, not to mention the offer, had come out of the blue. Sure, he had heard inklings of such a plan in the works, had even talked to an old friend from Phoenix who expected to be one of the people under consideration for its directorship. Robert figured he had been ruled out because of his choice to leave the FCI years ago. But somehow he stifled his incredulity, and found his voice.

"Stephen, I'm really flattered. Your offer does interest me. But what about the selection process? Don't you have to go through Civil Service recruitment and a quality assurance committee of some sort before making a selection?"

"Yes, there is such a process. But I'm sure you understand that I have a great deal of influence. I can assure you that my support and personal guidance will help the committee to make the right decision," Stephen answered with a hint of intrigue in his voice.

With that answer, Robert understood how the ballgame was being played. But he had never expected to participate. Business as usual. "Stephen, I need a few days to think about this. My wife was not very happy in Washington, and we've all settled in quite nicely down here. The kids are in top-notch private schools, and we've really woven ourselves into the social fabric."

Stephen knew well how unsociable the Gordons had become during Robert's previous tenure. They just didn't seem to fit in the "In" crowd at the Institute. Robert's wife seemed particularly uncomfortable with the wives' admittedly repetitive stories of their husbands' great accomplishments. But maybe they had matured a little. "Sure, think about it for a few days, but try to let me know one way or the other by the end of the week. I think you're the right man for the job, and I want to move quickly on this." Stephen was clearly signaling the end of the conversation. The director was a busy man.

"Thank you. I can assure you that I will consider your offer very seriously. On a scientific side, there is a great deal that I would like to do, and this will require resources. If the offer includes the ability to put together a team at my own discretion and to move rapidly into this new area, I would be inclined to accept." Robert had seen Mrs. Wendell Wilson on TV last week, expounding the glories of interferon, and knew of her "suggestion" that the FCI immediately allocate $50 million for interferon development. Was Stephen just cowtowing to her sudden interest?

"Robert, believe me, this is a very serious effort. I just learned last week that Congress has authorized $15 million of new money for fiscal 1981 to go into this program. So it is available today. And I have some flexibility in this year's budget that I can phase into the program. We will also initiate some new grants and contracts, as well as broaden our university support. I wouldn't be surprised to see this program reach $30 million annually in three years. We need a serious director for a serious program. This commitment includes a strong internal laboratory and clinical program under your personal direction. How about it?"

"I'll let you know by Friday."

"Fine, I'll have my administrative officer Fed Ex an offer letter. You know it won't be the official offer, since you have to go through the committees, but it will outline the resources and arrangements we plan to put on the line to develop this program. Will that help?"

"Absolutely. I look forward to receiving the letter, and I'll get back to you on Friday. And thank you, Stephen."

Robert agonized over the decision. As the week wore on, he was having trouble concentrating, running more and working less. Should he stay at home, where things were reasonably solid, conflicts aside? Mrs. Arthur T. Hastings, matron of Atlanta's second most prominent family, had committed herself and her considerable personal posture to his program in the Cancer Center. After all, he was a tenured professor. Although he worried some about Dennison, he was likely to become cancer center director. Once that occurred, he'd be permanently affixed to Mallory, something that he was sure would please his family. And the FCI offer had Stephen's trademark aura of uncertainty. If the promised resources failed to materialize, or, more likely, be there at the start and then gradually dwindle in favor of the long-established drug development effort, where would that leave Robert? Certainly, he couldn't assume his Mallory position would be held for his return.

An option was to depart Mallory under a six month leave of absence arrangement, keeping his options open in case Stephen had second thoughts down the road. Any longer than that and he knew his position would be usurped by one of the FCI-trained oncologists he had recruited to join him. One of them, an aggressive young man named Peterson, was the obvious candidate to take over the directorship. Peterson would hardly keep the position warm for his return if things didn't go smoothly at FCI. And Robert wasn't at all sure he wanted Peterson in his position -- the man was too diffuse in his approach to research, and his motives were unclear. Sometimes he seemed more interested in department politics and faculty wives than he did in pursuing his work. And patient care ranked low on his priority list.

But the numbers in Stephen's letter were nothing less than awesome to a man who had been fighting hard to get a $70,000 grant approved, and whose private research support amounted to barely $100,000 a year. Stephen had promised, in writing, $5 million to $6 million yearly in a directly controllable budget for the internal laboratory and clinic, plus $10 - $20 million in grant and contract support to administer. His entire annual budget for oncology at Mallory was a little over $1 million, and Robert had 35 people to support on it. It seemed he was on a treadmill, always trying to find another $10,000 or $20,000 to do this or that. Robert knew his immunology laboratory could never be "world class". Talent plus resources equaled world class science. If you lacked one of the two, talent was the least critical. Robert could see his interest in antibodies and toxin conjugates being passed over by those with resources he could never marshall here. The FCI offer would solve these problems.

He'd practically memorized the letter by now. "You will be the director of the Biotherapy Program with complete responsibility over hiring of new personnel, design of new laboratory space, and strategic program development. You will be an associate director of cancer therapy and work with minimal supervision. Although the usual personnel ceilings and controls are unavoidable, I can assure you that you will have broad latitude with respect to your budget, and I will see that position slots and space are made available for program development within those budget figures." The letter had been signed by Stephen's Administrative Officer.

He calculated that the $5 million or so would allow him to put into gear a program encompassing 30,000 to 40,000 square feet, with about 100 to 150 in personnel. Enough for a world class effort in developing biological substances for cancer treatment. And he was encouraged by the use of the new term "biotherapy". If it had been coined by Stephen, as he suspected, then it was further evidence of a true commitment, a brother to chemotherapy, Stephen's undisputed baby.

He'd do it.

Mary Margaret was more than mildly distressed. She too had been going through the decision process. And while she recognized the seriousness of the offer, she knew that she and the children could not be convinced to move back to Washington. Five years had been enough, much more than enough. They were happy and settled in Atlanta, and here they would stay.

But Robert could go. She knew what his career and his patients meant to him and wouldn't stand in his way. Anyway, she secretly suspected that he'd head up the program for a year or maybe two at the most, then run into the typical FCI roadblocks. Things couldn't have changed much in that regard over the past few years, and that man Musso was still pulling the strings. So if things worked out and Robert insisted the family permanently settle in the East, maybe she'd reconsider. But she wouldn't be at all surprised if he was back at Mallory within a year.

She had prepared a special southern dinner. His decision obviously made by the look of relief on his face. She'd put linen on the table, lit candles, and farmed the children out to the neighbors. They needed some peace and quiet to discuss their plans.

Robert, as usual, jumped right to the center of the issue. "MM, I want to go back and do this. The resources Stephen is offering are enormous. There'll never be another opportunity like this in my career. Just think of it! A $5 million annual internal budget, and $10 to $20 million of grant funds to administer. I just can't pass it by," Robert jabbered on enthusiastically.

She felt as if her heart was being pulled out of her. But she answered, "Yes, you go. I think you're right. This is indeed a tremendous opportunity. And our marriage is strong enough to survive long-distance, at least until you get a chance to feel the situation out."

"Are you sure you don't want to come with me? We'd have a nice house this time, no cramped apartments. And there must have been some staff turnover. Maybe the social scene wouldn't be so isolating."

"Yes, I'm quite sure. The children really need to stay in their current schools, and you know how much I love Atlanta." They were both silent for a few moments, looking at each other over their wine glasses.

"How often do you think you'll be able to come home?" Mary Margaret ventured, trying hard to keep from crying.

"Well, Washington to Atlanta is only a one hour flight. I'd like to get home every weekend, but finances might be a little tight," Robert began, introducing the topic that he had dreaded bringing up. "As you know, government salaries are not very good, particularly at the top end."

"How bad will it be?"

"Well, my guess is I will have to take a $20,000 yearly pay cut for this job. You may have to consider going back to work." Robert was having difficulty reading his wife's reaction. It looked as if clouds were passing over her face. He remained silent while she worked through his response.

Mary Margaret's gut reaction was anger -- she'd be losing a husband, at least part time, and gaining the responsibility of a job, and what went with it. She was 39 years old. Her life was in order. Children in the right schools and she was in the right social groups to pursue her personal goals. She was president of the Mallory auxiliary and was planning a program with the Atlanta Chamber of Commerce to develop a series of parks and recreational facilities around Memorial Hospital. A return to the daily grind of a job hadn't been in her plans. Robert took for granted all of the time and schedule shuffling necessary to manage a family and a house, not to mention her personal goals. Add on a job and an absent husband ... . But this was an incredible opportunity for him. And his work was so very important. Her decision was made.

"Robert, don't worry. I can go back to work. It won't be a problem. In fact, I just talked to Carolyn Johnson at the Coke Foundation, and they need a grants administrator. The same work I did during medical school. It would be perfect. It's from 9:00 to 3:30, so I can still be home for the children and to make dinner. The pay isn't great, but it'll help out, I'm sure. And if it means you can come home more often, I'll gladly do it."

Robert was visibly relieved. Mary Margaret seemed genuinely excited about returning to work. Maybe she should have done it sooner. Robert walked over and held her close. He felt that familiar tremble. "MM, I can't tell you how much your love and support mean to me. We can do it! Many couples couldn't, but we can! I love you, and I'll miss you and the boys terribly, but if we're both working, and I get back every other weekend or so, it won't be so bad. And if it all works out, maybe you'll be joining me soon."

Mary Margaret had her doubts about that. "Let's not kid ourselves. This is going to be a difficult separation, and even every weekend would not be the same as having you here every night, no matter how late. But, you clearly need to do this, and I know our family's internal ties are strong enough to sustain us. And if the long-distance bit doesn't work out, yes, I will come to Washington." She knew the permanent move wasn't realistic. Government pay would mean working in Washington, kids in public schools, small house and daily compromises. The thought of "East Coast life" nauseated her.

But she would do anything he asked, and they both knew it.

At 30,000 feet, life seems somehow uncomplicated. No telephone jangling, no visitors in and out of the office, the only interruption the flight attendant offering more of that godawful coffee. It was late 1980, and Robert was returning from the First International Hybridoma and Monoclonal Antibody Conference in San Francisco. Even though he was on government travel orders, stuffed in a middle seat and sweaty, he was having difficulty controlling his enthusiasm, and very nearly began babbling about antibodies to the man seated next to him, until he noted the salesman's catalog of bathroom fixtures. The college kid on his other side with rock music pounding into each ear probably wouldn't be interested either. So Robert put on his headphones and let his mind race over all he had heard.

He could already envision how these huge amounts of pure antibodies could be used to deliver drugs straight to the cancer cell, and away from healthy tissue. What a difference this could make in the toxicity of cancer treatment! If he could lessen side effects and increase effectiveness, standard chemotherapy would become obsolete overnight. He could barely wait to touch ground and get his team together, for he knew that this was hot scientific stuff indeed, and he must move both quickly and creatively.

Since Kohler and Milstein's development of hybridoma technology in Britain, monoclonals were being churned out with increasing rapidity and ease throughout the world. Although most were still of mouse origin, initial forays into human monoclonal antibody production were promising.

And the list was growing, daily it seemed, of previously out-of-reach biological substances, some only hypothesized to exist, being isolated more efficiently, and far more cheaply, than scientists had dared to imagine scarcely 2 years earlier. Just the names sparked excitement -- interferon, interleukin, colony stimulating factor, macrophage activating factor, tumor necrosis factor. Scientific meetings on immunology no longer consisted of conjecture; clear data was emerging on substances that had been only imagined.

At the conference, and in the animated conversations between talks, it was clear that most investigators were looking at the obvious -- direct use of single monoclonal antibodies in cancer therapy. But Robert was more far-sighted, realizing the intrinsic value of the spectacular specificity of the "magic bullets" in purification, diagnosis and treatment. Theoretically, monoclonal antibodies could be used not only to ferry toxic cargo to cancer cells, but could detect any infectious organism. The uses were almost limitless -- not only in human health care, but in veterinary medicine as well. Robert could envision combination chemotherapy loaded on antibody cocktails. "We've got plenty of toxic chemicals. We just need a better delivery mechanism, and antibodies will do it," he mused.

Robert looked out over the wing of the L1011. These coast-to-coast trips and the commuting from Washington to Atlanta were exhausting. He'd never been particularly afraid of flying, but did once in a while experience slight unease at the artificiality of sitting calmly in a multi-ton metal structure flying through the air at 30,000 feet. The familiar Chuck Yeager-like drone came on. "Ladies and gentlemen, we've been cleared for landing at Dulles International Airport. Please extinguish all smoking materials, and fasten your safety belts in preparation for landing. The weather is fine in Washington, and we anticipate a smooth trip down." These pilots, he thought, the world's greatest liars! If a wing falls off, the guy will say, "minor mechanical problems, folks. Relax and have a cocktail while we take her down for repairs." Going along at the old 30,000 was no sweat, but the ups and downs worried Robert. He distracted himself by going over the events of the past few months.

In the fall of 1980, Robert had accepted Stephen Musso's offer to head the new biotherapy program. And true to Stephen's word, the money rapidly flowed into the biotherapy program bank account. Robert had been interviewing and hiring scientists and technicians at a frenzied rate, and the laboratory space itself was in a state of renovation. Fortunately, Jim Banner, the contract program director, had been supportive in every way, and in fact he and Robert were already planning to collaborate on some immunotherapy projects. Banner's experiments were in animals, and Robert wanted to extend some of those ideas to humans. Jim was proving invaluable in getting the fledgling biotherapy program off and running, and their planned joint projects added an extra jolt of motivation. Plus, next week the new clinic and hospital wing would be open. Things were moving swiftly, and Robert was pleased.

Never before, he thought, had a world class scientific group been put together so rapidly. With the resources made available, Robert had immediately recruited 20 of the top Ph.D. cancer researchers from within the FCI and around the country. He had set up a broad program in monoclonal antibody production and the extraction of lymphokines from tissue culture. He had major plans for the large ACRC fermentation plant -- it was to be the factory for lymphokine and antibody production starting with no less than the magical-sounding alpha interferon.

Alpha interferon would very likely be the first genetically-engineered biotherapeutic for cancer. Robert already had patients lined up. Although alpha interferon had been fiddled with for several years following its discovery in the 1960s, it had been nearly impossibly expensive to produce by extraction, with estimates ranging up to $1 billion to procure sufficient amounts from blood-banks to carry out the kinds of clinical trials essential to see whether it might truly be efficacious in cancer treatment. Robert knew well that the entire FCI budget was barely $1 billion a year -- no one would even conceive of allocating such an all-encompassing chunk to pursue one substance, no matter how promising and how hyped up about it old Mrs. Moneybags Wilson was.

But genetic engineering had saved the day. And like monoclonal antibodies, it rendered current biological science, the extraction of interferon from blood bank blood cells, practically obsolete overnight.

In the 1970s, researchers had found ways to manipulate bacterial enzymes called restriction endonucleases as biochemical scissors of sorts. These restriction enzymes are normally summoned by a bacterium to hack up the DNA of invading viruses, while the bacterium's own DNA was protected by chemical groups. But these enzymes in the hands of researchers could be used to snip DNA, any DNA, at specific points. This allowed researchers to cut out the piece of DNA coding for a specific protein, stick it into a bug, and develop a factory producing the protein in a test tube.

The first success story had been insulin -- the molecular scissors snipped out the human insulin gene, which was then stuck into the genetic material of the common gut bacterium E. coli. The genetically engineered E. coli then churned out human insulin. It was human insulin and wouldn't evoke an allergic reaction in human diabetics as cow and pig insulin sometimes did. Growth hormone had come next. Genetic engineering was to biological science what the airplane was to transportation. It swooped down, and suddenly opened up possibilities in developmental therapeutics never before imagined.

And the elusive, rare proteins of the immune system were prime candidates for this new genetic engineering.

The landing, as promised, had been smooth, as was the short tram ride. Robert was now in his red Mazda RX-7, racing at 80 mph along the backroads of Virginia. His radar detector, illegal in Virginia, was neatly hidden behind the dashboard. As long as he knew where the police were before they knew where he was, he was in good shape.

Robert had good reason for his excitement. The initial dose of genetically-engineered alpha interferon would find its way into a cancer patient's body in his new facility next Monday. It was to be the first large-scale clinical trial of the substance, and the first of the 80 selected patients were already being prepped in the hospital. It would be an historical moment for his new program. Sure, M.D. Anderson had treated eight patients with it already, so technically they were first, but it would be his biotherapy program's trial which would set the pace for testing of similar genetically-engineered biologicals in years to come.

Although working with Genentech and Hoffman-LaRoche had been difficult, Robert had been able to negotiate the various hurdles and get the trial underway well ahead of three large university programs competing for this trial. There was nothing like the clout of the FCI to make things happen! It wasn't specifically stated anywhere, but the pharmaceutical companies knew that a positive FCI trial or two would pave the often rocky road to FDA approval, that final and most important hurdle to commercial success. With relatively little effort, and unhampered by the usual laborious FDA review and consent process, the first large scale trial with a genetically-engineered biological was underway at ACRC.

The airplane was soaring and Robert Gordon was the test pilot.

CHAPTER 15

CONTACTS

July 1, 1982

The phone jangled and, as usual, Robert jumped out of his seat. Damn that phone! He'd been griping about the air-raid like ring for months, but his government administrative officer could only be bothered to get things done between Tuesday noon and Thursday at 10:00 A.M., and then only with a ton of papers to be meticulously filled out. Government! It would probably take nothing less than a presidential order to get the phone taken care of.

Robert was actually grumbling out loud when he picked up the receiver. A sweet young voice began, "Dr. Gordon, please hold for Senator Daniels."

The foghorn voice that boomed over the line matched the ear-splitting ring. "Dr. Gordon, is this Dr. Gordon?" bellowed a rich Texas voice from Washington. "I need to talk to you about a friend of mine, a friend with cancer. Can you help me?"

Well, this one sure didn't waste any time. "Well, Senator, I don't know. I'll need a little more information. Can you have a medical report sent to me, or can you fill me in over the phone?" Robert answered patiently. He could field these calls in his sleep by now. He hadn't gotten one from the White House, yet, but he had received daily calls from the various Congressmen and their staffs. All, of course, wanting personal help from the FCI. He was even thinking about hooking up a special recorded message for them, because the conversations were always the same. "We're not trying to influence you in any way, just trying to see if there's anything available in your program." Well, sure, there was never overt influence, but when Robert didn't move with the speed the congressman thought was due him, it was not uncommon to receive a follow-up call from Stanley Lizzard or even Dr. Musso. They all knew on which side of the bread the butter was placed.

"He's a 55 year old man in good health, except he has this damned colon cancer," shouted the senator. "Can you cure him?"

Sure. They all wanted a cure. These were some of the most intelligent people in the country, able to handle billions in budgets and appropriations with ease. Yet their incredible naivete about medicine never failed to stun Robert. A two-sentence description of the patient, and he wants no less than a promise of a cure over the phone.

"Well, Senator, I don't know about a cure, but I'd be happy to have a look at the medical records or see your friend. Colon cancer is a tough problem, and we don't have any magic there. I can tell you that we've treated nearly 20 colon patients with this new form of interferon, and the results are not impressive. However, we are working on approaches using monoclonal antibodies ..."

"What's that? Monophonal whats?"

"A special type of immune system protein that we can use to attack cancer cells. Anyway, I'd be glad to see your friend, and determine whether he might be a good candidate for this new program."

"Okay, Dr. G., I'll relay the message. I just wanted to touch base and see if this was worth pursuing. His name is John J. Owens, and he's a fine, fine man. I want you to do everything you can to help him. Keep my office informed, and be sure to let me know if I can help in any way, understand?"

"Sure," Robert muttered. A trade of favors. "Okay, Senator, if his physician contacts me, I'll schedule a look at him. Good day," and he slowly placed the phone back in its cradle.

He hadn't mentioned it to the Senator, for it would only complicate things, but the powerful Mr. Owens was already well known at the Institute. He was an extremely rich man who had been funding research in colon cancer all over the country for the last several years. Robert didn't need to see the medical history. The man had colon cancer with a slow growing metastasis in the liver. Otherwise his general health was quite good, and in fact Mr. Owens ran 10 miles or more a day prior to his illness.

This was the second contact about Mr. Owens that had come directly to Robert. After a visit to his fermentation project, Roger Salla had called on him about three weeks ago to say that he had been approached by Mr. Owens and wanted to know how the interferon trials were looking. Roger had been targeted, Robert supposed, because of his hush-hush work on a colon cancer virus. Robert attempted to be upfront about the interferon work, and expected Roger to fill him in on the virus project in return. Wasn't exchange of ideas what science was all about?

"Well, Roger, the results with colon cancer using interferon don't look good. We have treated maybe 20 patients, and haven't seen a single response. Two patients had minor shrinkage, but nothing that I could call a true clinical response to treatment. These results are kinda discouraging."

"I'm not too surprised," Roger had answered, who'd always thought that interferon was a bunch of garbage. "We've looked at colon cancer cells in vitro, and they don't show any particular sensitivity to interferon. You know this is a tough tumor to kill with anything."

"True, although the rumor mill has it that you're making some progress in tracking down a causative virus. What's happening?"

Roger's voice had suddenly become more guarded, and he began fidgeting with the papers in his arms and looked at his watch. "Well, we have been working in this area, but have nothing to report as yet. We do, however, need a great deal of help from your colleagues in A." He glanced at his watch again, clearly uncomfortable.

Robert had had an idea what was coming. "In what way?"

"We need cells grown up in the fermentation plant. You know it takes a lot of cells to isolate a virus. I understand your program is using a good bit of the plant as well," Roger had ventured.

"Yes, we're using approximately 40% of the plant capacity to produce macrophage activating factor (MAF), a new lymphokine that might be very valuable in cancer treatment. But still, I understand that you are receiving a large number of cells on a weekly basis. Since we both obviously need the plant for priority work, I suppose the only solution is to get Stephen to expand the capability by building another one."

"Well, that's certainly a possibility, but not for the short term, and you know I need my cells now."

"But you're getting your cells. And I'm getting my MAF."

"But it's not enough." There was a long pause. Robert couldn't help but wonder where the needs of patients had gone in all of this. He and Salla were like two little kids fighting over the same sandbox. Shouldn't priorities be evaluated according to which project would serve patients first? Robert wondered uneasily just how far Roger would go. He didn't have long to wonder.

"Do you think you could stop producing your MAF for a few months, and let me finish this colon cancer cell production program?" Roger had the gall to ask next.

Robert's answer had been immediate. "No, no, we can't change our strategy on a moment's notice. And I'm not at all sure that such a change is even warranted. We are very close to isolating a substance with high biological activity for activating macrophages, and I think that the substance may prove very useful in treatment. We are projecting clinical trials by spring. Therefore, your program as well as mine has high priority. I think we'll have to proceed together, as we have been."

Roger had just shook his head. Gordon still didn't understand that Roger's words echoed Stephen's wishes. And with Stephen, Roger came first. Priorities, indeed. "Well Dr. Gordon, priorities can be changed. You'll see." And with that, he had turned the corner and left Robert in mid-sentence.

So when the second request to look into the Owens case came, Robert had been as cordial as he could. He knew he couldn't afford to rock the boat. He was still thinking over Salla's threat, and wondering whether the gears were already in place to cut back his program. So far Stephen's commitment to him had been honored, and over the first year every personnel position and every square foot of space had come through just as ticketed. And quickly. But over the last month or two, Robert had sensed some softening. Personnel actions were moving just a little bit slower. Tim had commented that there was considerable difficulty in bringing on board the last series of technicians, something about a government personnel ceiling. This hadn't been a problem over the past year, and Robert suspected that Stanley was tightening the strings a little, begin the choking process and see what happened. So the warning from Roger was indeed ominous. He just might be able to alter priorities, especially since he was in so solidly with Musso.

Robert knew that he must move full speed ahead while the going was good. If they intended to knife him, he wanted to be so far ahead that to do so would cut their own throats.

It was the weekly associate directors' meeting in Stanley Lizzard's plush office. The men directly under the Lizard were Jack Buerger for drug development, John Rogers for radiotherapy, Louis Brody for clinical oncology, David Ryan for surgery, Peter Green for cancer clinical trials, and Robert for biotherapy. These weekly gatherings in "The Lizard's Den", plus two or three weekly retreats a year, were used to allocate the Division's $160 million.

And it was a constant battle, each man tried to garner more support for his program. There was never enough money for drug development; radiotherapy required more and more expensive machines; clinical trials needed more money to fund clinical work at the universities; funding for a special project in surgery had to be immediate. David Ryan would typically be the first to get a request granted. Next to the Lizard, Roger Salla and Sam Fish, he was Stephen Musso's favored son.

On the rare occasion when a decision was actually made, it fell to Stanley to take it to the FCI executive committee. If they saw things in a different light, decisions that had seemed perfectly rational on Monday could be completely reversed on Tuesday. History which would support one point of view on Monday could be rewritten and altered by Tuesday. Because of these bizarre but frequent manipulations Robert coined the phrase "38 minute commitment". The FCI had the curious ability to say one thing one minute, and to change it the next, always on the pretext that the change was in the best interest of cancer research and the "public". And the practical impact could be enormous.

More than once, an academic scientist had been offered a position at the FCI, had notified his university, had even begun to move or actually arrived at the Institute, only to find that the job he had been offered had been "reallocated". In private industry, these sorts of actions would result in a legal battle. In the rational world, commitments couldn't be simply made and then yanked away. Not so for the government. The government couldn't be sued (unless they agreed to be sued), so there was little recourse for the victim, who was left in a "tough luck" situation. These sorts of changes were part of the very fabric of FCI life, an institution supposedly concerned with quality of life. So for the people who made up the venerable Institute, you took what you could get, never sure what was going to change -- and when.

This meeting was typical. John Rogers opened up the bickering.

"I've got to have more money for our new neutron therapy unit at the University of Southern California. We made a commitment to them three years ago to build this unit, and now it's time to write the check. Stanley, you know my budget was slashed at the last retreat, and I really don't know where this money is going to come from. We may need help from upstairs on this."

Stanley shot back, "What do you mean help from upstairs? This is something clearly within your program. You've got to take care of it."

"Stanley, you know that's impossible. You know my budget better than I do. We made the commitment, in writing, then the neutron generator was eliminated from my budget two years ago and was not reinstituted at our last retreat. I was told these funds would be reinstituted, and the program made commitments based on your assurance that there would be "no problem". Now, we're in a position of having the reactor half built, and it's time to pay the contractors and make good on our arrangement with the university," John responded passionately.

Stanley turned with obvious irritation to the DCT Administrative Officer. "What are the legalities here, Mike, do we have a firm contract with USC?"

Michael, the perfect government mind, cited chapter and verse of the arrangement, assigning a curt "yes" or "no" to every point, satisfying first what he thought Dr. Musso would want, next the Lizard, and finally his own need to look good and advance his GS rating. He could figure out a way to get around nearly everything. "Well, we do have a contract, but it has several outs."

"Such as?" Stanley prompted.

"Funding could occur in fiscal '82 or calendar '82. We were intentionally unclear about that language when we wrote the contract. Thus, we have several months of flexibility left. Plus, certain performance criteria are specified in the contract. Perhaps these haven't been met. Hence, if we want to leave the neutron generator half finished, we could come back to USC and say they didn't meet these commitments. Finally, I've had some confidential discussions with USC administrative people myself, and they may come up with some private funding to complete the project. Therefore, I do not totally agree with Dr. Rogers' point of view. I think there are other ways to skin this cat."

Rogers was out of his seat, sputtering, "But, but, but, you just told me two days ago that you felt there was a commitment under this contract, and that we intended to honor it. How could it all have changed?"

Stanley interceded. "Hold it, hold it. Don't get excited. We'll somehow get this generator up, but John, you must understand that this could take several years. Mike is simply stating that we have some flexibility in this matter. Now let's go on to other deliberations for the moment, and we'll come back to this within the next week or so."

Robert silently chalked up yet another 38 minute commitment. It didn't matter whether it was a box of paper clips that cost a quarter, a personnel action that cost a few thousand dollars, or a neutron generator for three quarters of a million dollars. Government could, and did, make and break commitments anytime it wanted to. Human costs aside, FCI made the rules.

Robert knew the source of this particular problem. The $750,000 for the neutron generator had been chewed up in new drug development centers, the grand new program initiated by Stephen and Stanley, who would now try to pry more funds loose from Congress by citing the plight of USC. Perhaps the Congressman from California could be of assistance. It was an interesting balance that had to be struck -- you needed to make things look bad enough to need their help, but you simultaneously needed to demonstrate the high-level of the FCI commitment -- even if it meant fixing a few budget numbers. Convinced, the targeted Congressman would then make his series of telephone calls pressing Stephen and calling the head of the FCI Congressional budget committee. Ultimately, a hasty investigation would show a need for three neutron generators, none of which the "overburdened" FCI could fund. With any luck, that would bring more money from Congress, a little special allocation. And once again, Stephen had effectively re-routed radiotherapy money into drug development. After all, it was for a good purpose, to fight cancer.

With the neutron generator dilemma temporarily shelved, attention turned to another area that could be eaten away, like a cancer, Robert thought bitterly, to make more room for drug development. Biotherapy. He was shaken from his reverie by a nudge from Jack Buerger on his right. It was his turn.

"Robert, I understand you have some difficulties in the fermentation plant. Can you bring us up to date on what's happening there?" asked Stanley.

Robert straightened, and explained that he wasn't the one with a problem. He outlined the current programs and budgets of the ACRC fermentation plant, and concluded "we're using about 40% of plant capacity, and Roger is using about 60%. Our 40% is going toward the production of MAF, interferon and various other lymphokines and cytokines that may be very useful in cancer treatment within the next two years. Roger's component is directed toward the mass production of three colon cancer cell lines that I understand he is using for putative virus isolation. Of course, we don't know exactly what he's using these cells for because the project has been somewhat circumspect. However, it is my understanding that this production is high priority and must go on." There, that's what he wants to hear.

Stanley smiled, but not because he was satisfied. Robert was still so naive. "High priority" -- what an understatement. In truth, it was whatever Roger wants, Roger gets, and that had been true for several years. Since Stephen had become director, he had steered much of the flexible resources towards Roger's laboratory, and Stanley was about to do more of the same.

"Robert, the executive committee met last week, and a decision was made about your program. Now, I know you are going to disagree with this, but you must understand that this represents a high level decision. These fellows thought it was in the best interest of the Institute and the public we serve. We've decided to reallocate the fermentation plant 80% viral oncology, 20% biotherapy. I hope you can live with this figure, although I know it will be difficult. Please, reorient the program with viral oncology and see that things are made to fit within that specification.

My God, thought Robert, that bastard Salla knew all about this when he made his threat! Now he looked directly into the squinty eyes of Stanley's sharply-cut face. The man was clearly taking a pathological pleasure in all of this. The two men had never liked each other, but now the tension between them was noticeable, palpable, to everyone in the room.

Robert tried hard to corral his outrage before he spoke. He knew he must play the game, but he just couldn't swallow this obvious breach of commitment. So he blurted out, "Stanley, this is a major mistake. I don't care where the decision came from, nor how the committee reached its decision, but the production of MAF should be very, very high priority, and I think Roger, very frankly, has plenty of cells to do his research. Has this sacred committee completely forgotten about cancer treatment? About patients? This looks to me like a simple power play to take over more of the fermentation plant capacity, and to glorify Roger, not solve a scientific problem. Can you, or anyone for that matter, bring us up to date on the uses of these precious cells, and the reasons why they decided to reallocate the fermentation capacity toward a higher level for Roger? Don't we deserve a rationale for such a decision?"

Stanley found these questions intensely irritating. Robert knew how the game was played and he knew those questions just weren't to be asked, yet he continued to pry into FCI decision-making. Everyone at the table knew that such things were never questioned, never even discussed. The Executive Committee, read that Musso, was tantamount to Mount Olympus, and that was that. Would the man never learn?

Stanley responded slowly, as if Robert was some dim-witted child. "All I can tell you is that the executive committee in general, and Dr. Musso in particular, said that they had reviewed Dr. Salla's need for more cells, and it was clear to them that these requirements were higher priority than the production of MAP."

"That's MAF," Robert interrupted.

"Whatever. If you want further review of the facts, you will have to discuss it directly with Dr. Musso." With that, Stanley stood, and, like at a Presidential news conference, it was clear that the meeting was over. But not for Robert. He also stood, and tried to continue the debate as the group exited -- another mistake.

"Stanley, I do need to talk to Stephen about this one. This represents a clear deviation from the commitment he made to me in 1980. It's not just another neutron generator. I feel strongly that I should have been consulted about this before the decision was made. I will speak to him."

"Well, you can make your own appointment, but it's my view that it's not going to do you any good, and may very well do you long-term harm. The fight simply isn't worth it. Leave it alone."

"I hear you, but I can't proceed until I settle this. There is a matter of principle here, can't you recognize that?" Robert almost pleaded.

"Principle! What the hell are you babbling about? We're talking about things that the director wants done. If you keep standing on your ridiculous principles, you'll wind up with your ass in a sling," Stanley shot back, stomping down the hall.

Robert knew it was hopeless, but he had to have at least some say. He'd speak to the almighty Musso. And soon.

The phone was ringing obnoxiously when Robert returned from lunch, a few days after the meeting in Stanley's office that had set into motion the slashing of his fermentation program. On the other end was none other than the Lizard himself.

"Robert, we need to talk about a patient."

Robert was piqued by Stanley's unusual use of the word "patient". The man wouldn't know a patient from an ant hill. Someone must be pushing his button again.

"Yes, Stanley, what is it?"

"I've been contacted by Representative Hampton about a man from Connecticut who he thinks you might be able to help. His name is Mr. Weil, and he's an 80-year-old case with lung cancer."

"This case has had done all that can be done in New York. He has been through Sloan-Kettering and has repeatedly failed chemotherapy, after failing radiotherapy. They're looking for a new approach -- how does the interferon data look?"

Talk of patients and new approaches distracted Robert from his immediate political problems. "Not very promising for lung cancer, I'm afraid to say, Stanley. We've treated more than 30 patients and seen only one partial response, a patient with a slow-growing adenocarcinoma. I'm not encouraged."

This just further confirmed Stanley's lack of faith in interferon, or any biological. However, that had nothing to do with this particular situation. Mr. Weil was an important industrialist and a very influential man, and these matters made a difference in Congress. He needed whatever services the FCI could provide, even if there was no scientific basis for them. He would come to the Institute and be assured that whatever was newest would be tried on him. Robert had no choice.

"Well, you know how much I want to help these cases, and I want you to do whatever you can for Mr. Weil. Please arrange for an appointment so you can see him and encourage him to try interferon. Even if it doesn't work, it'll give him something to fix on in the short term," Stanley directed.

"But, Stanley, I don't think that would be possible. I'll be glad to see Mr. Weil and do what I can to help, but he won't be eligible for the interferon treatment because we have already filled all the slots in that protocol for lung cancer. Besides, he is not eligible based on age."

There was momentary silence on the other end. Stanley just couldn't believe that the brilliant Dr. Gordon could be so maddeningly thick.

"Maybe you didn't understand me, Robert. You are being told to treat Mr. Weil with interferon."

"But it will be a waste of time. And his slot, which doesn't, as I've pointed out, exist, could be used for someone who might truly benefit."

"That is not the point, goddamit. You've got to stop resisting the obvious. This must be the fifth time I've told you this in the last six months. When one of these cases comes along, and I call you, it is because it is important for you to respond appropriately. I repeat, I want Mr. Weil put on the interferon treatment, one way or the other, and if it's not done, you're going to be in even more hot water than you're already in."

Robert knew full well what Stanley meant. He had indeed been to Musso's office, and they had had a "forthright and candid discussion" of the biotherapy program and Robert's needs. As expected, the fermentation issue had been resolved 80% Salla, 20% Gordon. In addition, Musso had told Robert in no uncertain terms that he had to become more cooperative and work more in concert with his other division directors. Musso gave high marks to being a "team player."

The man had been adamant. "Over and over, Robert, I keep hearing of incidences in which you haven't cooperated. First from Jack Buerger, then Lou and Peter. These little frictions just cannot continue. We are a team here, a family, and if you can't fit in, then we'll have to make some new arrangements. I've given you a great deal in the last two years, and I expect performance on your part, not only in carrying out the biotherapy program, but in integrating it by responding to the needs of the Institute -- as they are articulated by this office. When Stanley gives you information on the executive committee's decision, I don't want any further questioning. That tends to be disruptive and causes difficulties for the other associate directors. And your attitude is influencing others. The other day, John Rogers was in here pressing me about his neutron generator funding. I think this move was a direct result of your discussion on the fermentation plant. You're disrupting our activities, and it must stop."

And Robert knew the underlying cause of the problem -- the attention his program was getting. He had been the subject of several media reports and television interviews, and there was even a book in progress about the work of the program. This kind of attention, and the success of interferon in treating certain kinds of leukemias and lymphomas, was bothering Stephen and Stanley, who could not directly take the credit publicly. Arlington was doing too well, getting too much credit.

The successes were indeed beginning to pile up. The interferon program put nearly 100 patients on trial in one year, an unprecedented number for a Phase I/II trial. A typical new drug trial would place maybe 15 patients on study in a year, and here, at a small program at Arlington, they had managed to more than quadruple the usual number. In addition, the study had been done quickly, efficiently, and had been presented to major scientific audiences and in a prestigious medical journal. Worse yet, these successes were attracting public inquiries, media attention and some congressional interest. This tended to bring further attention to the Arlington biotherapy program. Roger Salla's need for cells, real or not, was a convenient mechanism for Stephen to begin to choke Robert.

It was clear that Robert's successes were beginning to bother his superiors, so he knew he had to tread carefully on this latest request from Stanley, which of course meant for Stephen. "Sure, I'll be happy to see Mr. Weil, and if you insist, we will attempt to revise the interferon protocol to include five more patients. This and an age change will allow Mr. Weil to be treated, and us to stay within our approvals by the Institutional Review Board."

"Robert, do it any way you like, but get it done." And Stanley slammed down the phone.

CHAPTER 16

SUCCESS MEANS FAILURE

September 1982

It all started with a cow's eyeball.

A minor presentation at the cancer therapy board of scientific counselors meeting; an investigator from Utah with some information on a tumor in cattle. The tumor was not of economic interest to the cattle industry, but was a model for immunotherapy. The researcher was injecting the eye tumor with bacillus Calmette-Guerin (BCG), a bacterium known for some 20 years to be effective treatment for some animal cancers. BCG was one of a number of bacterial extracts which sometimes seemed to boost immunity, part of what was dubiously called "non-specific immunotherapy." In fact, BCGs on-again off-again activity had caused many of the problems that had put the whole field into disrepute in the early 1970s. And here it was again, presented to the board by Dr. Cliner.

Cliner was continuing the work of a colleague at the University of Utah who had recently committed suicide. Whether this drastic action was a reflection of the man's deep frustration at being unable to secure funding for what he truly believed was a worthwhile cancer treatment approach was of course unknown, but many believed he just couldn't fact another rejection.

The Utah BCG grant had recently received another horrible priority score, something in the 300s, when a funded study needed a score well under 200. Despite this mediocre scientific review, a second evaluation was called for which confirmed the previous peer review, recommending not funding the grant.

Subsequently, the grant that normally would be out of the system after one review, found itself on the desk of Robert Gordon, for yet a third review. To the ever-logical Robert, it didn't make much sense -- twice rejected, now submitted to him. So he simply assumed he was being called in because the work was a piece of history in the ill-fated area of immunotherapy, a field that was now being rejuvenated in the biotherapy program. Because no explanatory letter accompanied the submission, he thought the Institute just needed another professional point of view. And he did know quite a bit about BCG.

Robert simply didn't appreciate the depth of the considerations in this particular case, the meaning of this unprecedented third appeal. Had he been as expert in assessing the FCI political climate as he was in his chosen field of medicine, he might have averted yet another confrontation.

The fact was that the peer review system on which scientific quality is supposedly based meant very little to the outspoken Senator Haller from Utah, a man who had been instrumental in getting major radiotherapy equipment allocated to his state, not to mention various public reclamation projects, dams, and several public works endeavors, all to help Utah prosper and compete. And now he wanted to secure this BCG project - whether it made scientific sense or not.

Haller was, at the moment, heading a committee to investigate FCI management practices. And the perceptive and powerful man did business the old fashioned, government way, undercover. Behind the scenes arrangements served him well, keeping him out of the limelight, and getting effective actions for his state without political backwash. He was intrigued by the awesome FCI budget of over a billion dollars. Wasn't that of keen interest to the American people? Haller certainly thought so. Already Stephen Musso, Sam Fish, Stanley Lizzard and Roger Salla had testified before his committee. These men were instrumental in making the costly FCI decisions, and

Senator Haller wanted them on record with respect to the management of their respective programs.

Meanwhile, the FCI, particularly the chemotherapy development program, was taking quite a beating by the press. It was not a time to insult a powerful Senator. The Washington Post was running a major series investigating allegations of unreported toxicities from certain new drugs, especially in children, which always heightens interest. Two reporters, Rupp and Newfield, were busy snooping about the Institute, and indeed, they had uncovered the transfer of drugs from the FCI to certain university programs in violation of proper procedure and drugs transmitted from universities to individual physicians without proper controls and paperwork. The pharmacy logs were not in place, and various other irregularities were found. The Georgetown University program run by Paulo Brisella was particularly suspect. Paulo had been at the FCI for many years, and there seemed to be a strong flow of investigational drugs to Georgetown, more so than to any other university, and some of these drugs were arriving at the Georgetown pharmacy without proper requisitions, protocols or FDA approval. The reporters were on to something, a local story with national importance, and they meant to make the most of it.

And so Robert Gordon failed to see the big picture, how his decision might affect the political climate. What he saw was a question of the scientific merit of a project that had been reviewed, and rejected, time and again. He should have seen the project in the context of the inquisitive and powerful Senator from the same home state as the BCG investigator, coupled with the bad press from the Washington Press.

The confusing barrage of questions that Robert faced when delivering and explaining his rejection of the grant to the review board would have alerted a more suspicious person. First, he was subjected to a series of questions concerning the reasons for this third review of a rather small grant, which he couldn't answer. But he did maintain, over and over, that he felt the request should not be funded because the work was of a historical nature, and offered nothing new. Still, he was asked the same questions, as if the board wasn't sure that he really meant what he said. When Robert explained point by point where the proposal fell short, he thought he was telling them what they wanted to know.

But in a bizarre turn of events towards the end of the deliberations, Stanley Lizzard made the astounding suggestion that Dr. Cliner's work be resubmitted to a special committee and that his grant might be subdivided into two components for a final evaluation. And the board, who had just listened intently to Robert's affirmation of the shoddy science, went right along with Lizzard's suggestion. A new peer review committee would be formed to review for a fourth time Dr. Cliner's proposal. Case closed.

After the board meeting, Stanley called Robert to the side. "What the hell is wrong with you now? Didn't you understand that Stephen wanted that grant reviewed less contentiously? You didn't have to give a highly favorable review, no one's asking you to compromise your scientific reputation, but we did expect at the very least a neutral stance. You've really screwed up this time, Gordon."

Robert was stupified. "Stanley, I was asked to review this grant based on the science. No one intimated otherwise, and even had it been suggested that I review it differently, that would not have been acceptable. The science of this grant has been reviewed by three different groups, and all are in agreement, it simply doesn't pass muster. What has happened to standards around here? I see no reason for the constitution of yet another review committee, or the submission of a new grant proposal. But I supposed there were other reasons for that."

"Yeah, like why the hell don't you get your head out of your journals and open up a newspaper once in a while? You're damn right there are other reasons, although you're a little late in catching on. You'd better hope that your innocent views aren't transmitted upstairs. You're already in some hot water, and my advice is not to get in any deeper." Stanley stalked off down the hall.

Robert walked slowly towards the elevator. Our precious peer review system! Yet another committee designed to administer a decision, a prescribed course of action. What was it this time, Robert wondered -- something about Utah...

Robert sat in the outer office of the director, distracted from the latest New England Journal of Medicine by Melody, the most attractive GS-14 he had ever seen. Auburn hair down to her shoulders, large green eyes, a skirt right at the knees and a well-fitted sweater. She exuded a curious combination of efficiency and intelligence, and subtle sexuality. Watching her move gracefully around the office, supervising the GS-13s stimulated him a little for what was to come.

Half an hour later, Robert was finally summoned into the inner sanctum. Stephen rose from behind his huge shiny desk and motioned Robert to the casual furniture arrangement in the corner. "Sit down Robert. I want to talk to you," said Stephen in a flat, matter-of-factly-don't-waste-too-much-of-my-time-tone. No handshake, no casual talk, no war stories.

"Over the last two years we've had several conversations in this office. I've tried to help you understand how to work best as an FCI executive. You've done a good job in pulling your program together using the resources available. You've put together a credible scientific team and published well. However, you've failed miserably in understanding our processes and responding to the sensitivity of certain issues. And here you are again."

Robert suspected what was coming. Something to do with the Cliner affair, no doubt, and who knew what else.

"I've responded to the board's recommendation that a special review committee be set up for Dr. Cliner's grant. In fact, he is submitting two grants, splitting his work up for easier review. I am hopeful that this committee will act favorably on his proposals." And Stephen briefly outlined precisely what this committee would do. All of the individuals on it, unlike the thick-skulled Gordon, would know that on the surface they were to compromise an objective peer review group -- but one that was to turn in a positive response. This was never written down anywhere, not even specifically articulated, but it was absolutely understood. Dr. Cliner's grant would be funded, and perhaps a few other favors done. And this would lessen the pressure from the Haller committee on the investigation into FCI management. Senator Haller would be announcing the committee's findings pretty soon, and the Washington Post snoops were practically salivating in anticipation. Proper action on the Cliner grant would safeguard the FCIs, and Stephen's, reputation.

"Robert, I spent nearly six months getting this damn Cliner grant reviewed and reconstituted. I've practically written the thing myself. The decision of the board was a formality. All you were to do was to agree with the need for re-review, but, on being questioned, you took a hard negative stance, directly against my six months of groundwork bringing it through the system," Stephen said angrily.

"But it was never, never made clear to me that the review was anything other than a science review. I gave my honest opinion of it," Robert Sputtered.

"You're confusing honest reviews with the more subtle problem of emphasis. Had you merely said that you agreed with the previous reviews, but that there was room for rewriting with subsequent review, then everything would have been fine. Instead, you took the podium and really banged away at Dr. Cliner, his science, his grant, and the review process. That was unacceptable," Stephen snapped.

Robert sat there, going over the events in his mind once again. Well, maybe he had somewhat been outspoken, but BCG had already been evaluated many times and in multiple ways, and what Dr. Cliner was proposing just didn't come up to what he had though were FCI scientific standards.

But Stephen wasn't done. "I'll tell you this, Robert, and I want it not to go beyond this office. I want to be very clear. You need to get my messages, directly or indirectly, for taking affirmative action when I deem it necessary. Sometimes I'll tell you exactly what I need, and other times the message may come through Stanley, Michael or Sam. But however it comes, you must be sensitive and listen, then respond appropriately. If you have questions as to your expected course of action, consult with Stanley. That's what he's there for."

Robert stood up, anxious to leave, but Stephen signaled him to sit. "And while we're on the topic, I want to reiterate my comments concerning the matter of the fermentation plant. When I want to change priorities, and the executive committee issues such a ruling, I don't want their decisions rediscussed at the division level. It presents an improper influence on the other associate directors. Now, is that understood?"

Robert paused before he answered, trying to hold his astonishment, frustration and anger in check. "Well, yes, it is perfectly clear now. But our conversation is very disturbing to me and to be frank, I'm not sure that I can continue to work here if this is to be the arrangement. In coming back here to run the biotherapy program, I thought that you wanted a rapidly developed, scientifically credible effort, and I've tried my best to do that. Perhaps, I've been less sensitive to political issues than you'd like me to be, but, to be sure, I'll always respond to questions, any questions, directly and honestly. I cannot change that."

Stephen rose and walked toward the door, and Robert followed. "I understand your forthrightness. But perhaps a little compromise is what is needed. Surely you can be sensitive to political matters and still run your program. Give our conversation some serious thought. I don't want to have to go through this again with you." With that, and in full view of the GS-13s scurrying about, Stephen put out his hand, patted Robert on the back, and the interview was finished.

As Robert headed out of the enormous office, Melody handed him a package. "This is very important, from Dr. Musso. Something to do with a patient, I think," she said smiling.

"Thanks Melody," Robert stammered, still somewhat in shock from Stephen's tongue-lashing -- but not enough so that he didn't notice Melody's perfume. Shalimar.

Robert looked through the package in the elevator. The medical records of Senator Robert Tomasi, one of the more celebrated people to recently seek "special help" at the FCI. Everyone knew of Senator Tomasi and his plight. The fast-rising young Senator from Connecticut was compared often to John F. Kennedy -- good looking, brilliant, from an influential family, yet a man of considerable personal magnetism. He had been headed straight for the Presidency when the lymphoma arose. Of the one million people diagnosed with cancer each year, those with lymphoma were considered, at least by the oncologists to be "lucky." At least they could be treated, some could be cured, and a life expectation of ten years or even more was quite likely.

But for a potential President, even a ten year future was unacceptable. The leader has to appear indestructible. Just the word cancer, which struck paralyzing fear into many people, would doom any campaign, despite the man's exceptional record in two terms in the Senate. And in a 50 year old, it was particularly upsetting.

So Senator Tomasi sought not just an effective short term treatment, nor even a long term disease control. He wanted nothing less than a cure. He had even said in a much talked about television interview that treatment of his lymphoma came first, and that he would not run again for what was now the senior senatorship from Connecticut. First the cure, then he'd get his political agenda back on track.

Robert read the material over carefully. A nodular, poorly-differentiated lymphocytic lymphoma, a lot of long words meaning a slow growing clone of malignant lymphocytes. Immediately Robert's highly-trained brain began to tick off the drugs -- Chlorambucil and Prednisone; Cytoxan, Vincristine and Prednisone; Bleomycin, Adriamycin, Cytoxans, Oncovin and Prednisone; known as CP, CVP, and BACOP in the alphabet soup of chemotherapy. Tomasi had already responded well to CP, and now that his doctors were thinking of progressing beyond to another drug regimen, perhaps to bone marrow transplant. The Senator was talking about monoclonal antibodies, an approach still unfamiliar to many physicians, let along laypeople. But as a member of the Senate Science and Technology Committee, Tomasi was quite familiar with genetic engineering and molecular biology, and knew well the potential of monoclonal antibodies in cancer treatment, particularly lymphoma. He wanted to come to the FCI, or go to Stanford and have antibodies made against his lymphoma cells. And possibly try some interferon while he was at it.

Robert was intrigued by the Senator, a man who was bright, direct and honest, unusual characteristics for a politician, he thought. In fact, Senator Tomasi was very much like Robert himself. The Senator had been forthright against pork barreling and other forms of political favoritism, particularly the use of state and federal government by politicians for their own purposes. But now Senator Tomasi was faced with a dilemma -- should he use the government cancer treatment capability to fight his cancer, using his influence to gain privileged access, so that he could continue to be an honest leader? Would his ends justify his means?

Thinking back to his meeting with Stephen, Robert thought he had a pretty good idea of how Senator Tomasi must feel.

Stanley Lizzard and Louis Brody were talking over beers at Bruno's, a cozy restaurant where more business was conducted than in any of the FCI conference rooms. Investigators from all over the world met at Bruno's, and you could practically smell the political intrigue and influence above the aroma of pizza.

Lizzard loved Bruno's; being there, and more importantly, being seen there, made him feel important. And what he had to say to Brody really was important.

"Lou, I've heard through the grapevine that you're having some difficulty in getting patients to participate in the trials of those three new chemotherapeutic drugs Stephen wants us to test. What seems to be the problem? We've never lacked for volunteers before."

"It's the program, Stanley. I've been whipping my staff right and left to fulfill Stephen's wishes and get patients to sign up for those drugs, but the word's out. The drugs just don't work very well and they're highly toxic. The patients open up the newspaper or turn on the TV and learn about the wonders of interferon, lymphokines and monoclonal antibodies, and that's what they want."

"I was afraid of this..."

"And it goes deeper than that. I'm having a hard time getting the new clinical associates to understand that the drug studies must come first. It is a problem, and it's going to get worse."

"Well, Stephen thinks he has an answer and I wanted to get your feelings, since you've directly encountered the problem."

"Increase funding to biotherapy so that more people can participate? How will that make the drug studies seem more attractive?" Lou asked a trifle fearfully. He didn't like the ACRC competition one bit.

"No, in fact just the opposite. The root of the problem, both short term and long term, is that the biotherapy program is getting too damn much attention. Stephen's afraid that the national publicity may have negative implications for our main clinical programs here in Washington. He wants the process slowed down."

Lou looked visibly relieved. "Well, I'm certainly glad to hear that. But how will you do it? Scientifically, Gordon's doing a fine job, and the press seems to love him. He is rather good, you know. Did you see him on the local news last week? It's not his fault that "interferon" sounds so sexy, or that he is so photogenic."

"If he wants to be a media star he doesn't belong here. Anyway, Stephen has a plan."

"I rather thought he might..."

"Let's have Gordon come down and give a couple of seminars in Washington. This will heighten the fear on the part of our senior investigators that he is going too fast. He'll give one of his usual aggressive presentations saying that biotherapy is going to be very effective in cancer treatment. Replace chemotherapy, radiation and surgery. You know, The Fourth Modality and all that. You know the way he can charm the paint off the walls. But our researchers, devoted to drugs, won't be swayed, and they'll go after him. They'll put the pressure on, and he'll feel it. You know he's a sensitive, almost paranoid sort, too honest for his own good."

"Sounds fine, but will that be enough to get us back in the limelight?"

"No. We'll also slow down approval of his new protocols through the Washington Institutional Review Board. He'll probably continue to get his quick approvals through the Arlington IRB, but not here. Specifically, he has one monoclonal antibody program up and running, but he has a whole series of protocols using antibodies tagged with drugs and isotopes, that I don't want to go through the system. Those studies need to be done so that we can take the credit when the time comes. I am beginning to believe these approaches may be useful."

"I agree," Lou responded. "We've begun to look into conjugated monoclonals, too, and I think that's the way out of this box. Drug development has produced a lot of toxic chemicals. If we can just deliver them to the tumor site better, they may be useful and validate the money being spent here. And we've been evaluating new chemotherapeutics for far longer than Gordon's been fiddling with his biologicals. I say let's concentrate our antibody linked to drugs and isotope studies here in Bethesda."

"You're absolutely right, and that's what we'll do. But first, let's put the brakes on Gordon."

The five scientists and eight technicians jumped about the medium-sized office of their superior like little kids just told they are going to the circus. One in particular, Morgan Staley, pranced about hugging people at random, babbling "we've done it! we've done it!" to anyone who would listen, including the tank of fish. Robert looked them all over, a silly grin on his face too, and wondered fleetingly about Morgan's mental stability. He would plunge into a profound depression when the work wasn't going as he had anticipated, but he would also have these contagious fits of glee when things went well. He must be awfully hard to live with. The contagious giggling continued, because no one could think of a word to describe just how well things had gone.

"My God, do you realize we've taken the whole process through from start to finish!" Staley shouted. "We've made the antibodies, cured the human tumors growing in mice, we've killed the cancer cells in the test tube, and now we've produced the antibody for use in patients, and we've done it all in record time!"

"Not only that," added Robert, "but we've treated the first series of patients and proven beyond a doubt..."

"Absolutely," interrupted Staley, "proven that those antibodies actually find the cancer cells. It was amazing. Those nodules lit up like Christmas trees. The antibodies were all over the tumor cells and not on the normal cells at all. It really works! It almost blew my eyes out when I saw that under the microscope for the first time," babbled Staley, still jumping about the room.

"Let's get back to planet Earth" said Robert, not wanting to spoil the party, but trying to keep things in perspective. "The patients have not -- yet, shall I venture -- shown a tumor response, but ..." Half a dozen voices interrupted to finish the sentence "we all know what comes next. Yes, hook the antibody to a toxic substance, and repeat the series of experiments." Robert began chalking the protocols on the board.

"We will take iodine 131 and perhaps iodine 123 and hook them to antibody. Maybe also Abrin chain A toxin. Then later maybe try some chemotherapeutic drugs. Targeted drug therapy will really happen. And much sooner than anyone thought possible." And very much sooner than the brass in Washington thought possible, Robert mused silently.

"When can we get started? Soon?" asked Dr. Staley, like a little kid wanting candy at the circus.

"Well, I'm not sure when. It's true we have this contract with Conjugation Technology on the West coast, and we clearly have the ability to conjugate a variety of substances to the antibody. But our protocol approval process is slowing us down. They go before the IRB next month, which shouldn't be a problem, and then the Washington IRB. After the approvals are in place, we can start the conjugated antibody studies in patients, probably by this summer."

It was an exciting time in molecular biology, particularly long overdue for immunology, but the constant red tape was incredibly frustrating. Just a decade ago the immunologists worked in a black box, only able to hypothesize the existence of certain chemicals, then only able to obtain them by laborious extractions from donated tissues. But now there were three types of genetically engineered interferon, macrophage activating factor, new lymphokines such as interleukin-2, and the cell separator to remove lymphocytes from a patient, activate them in laboratory flasks, then reinfuse them. The possible applications of monoclonal antibodies were nothing short of mind-boggling. Biotherapy was expanding far more rapidly than anyone, even Robert Gordon, had imagined.

However, a nagging doubt was beginning to take root in the back of his mind. The science was here -- but could he count on consistently getting the FCI to translate these substances to patients quickly enough or would the political problems get in the way? What of the growing power play between the chemotherapy development program in Washington and biotherapy in Arlington? Robert realized that he was caught in the middle. If chemotherapy successes from Washington didn't parallel his successes with biotherapy, his program would ultimately be swallowed up by the larger component of the FCI. Musso could hardly stand by and watch him receive all the attention, while the drug work faded into the background. The undeniable facts were that the money, political power, and Stephen Musso were in Washington. And the positive results had to come from there, too.

Winter 1982

It wasn't at all usual for the executive committee of the FCI to meet to discuss the latest issues of National Geographic, Time, and the Washington Post. But when Dr. Gordon smiled back from the pages, it was a different story altogether.

If Gordon's superstar status in the press wasn't enough, he had recently made a much talked about major presentation at the American Cancer Society headquarters in New York. That had started the Wilson Committee whispering. The influential Mrs. Wilson was quite pleased at the unexpected rapid pace of the biologicals program over the past two years and there was talk of increasing appropriations. The spotlight was clearly on Dr. Gordon. And so the subject of the executive committee meeting on that cold winter day was the "Gordon problem."

Sam Fish began. "Well, we have been successful in getting rid of Jim Banner as the director of the Biolab Contract program. His criticism of our contracting process was just too much to tolerate. We fiddled with the contract and held discussions with Biolab. They agreed to get him transferred off site into a new institute set up by the company. He seems to be happy with the arrangement. The new man is in our pocket and should present no problems. We've also changed scientific management there with my appointment as FCI Director for ACRC."

"In the past six months, I have begun the reorientation of the Arlington contract programs to better serve our needs here in Washington, paring down their independent research program so that they function more as support for us. For example, George Trumpey's lab -- you all remember George, he's now at Oncos, Inc., in Palo Alto, and very satisfied, I might add -- has been integrated with Roger Salla's here in Washington. The contract research program has been cut by 50 percent, forcing the best of ACRC scientists to go elsewhere. Next was the transfer of the fermentation plant totally to Dr. Salla's, rendering it unable to produce new substances for biotherapy. We've done that.

Our next and most important task, as I'm sure you are all aware, is to restructure the biotherapy program. Stanley? Can you give us your thoughts, since you are the closest to our media darling, Dr. Gordon?" Fish sat down with a look of sublime satisfaction on his face. He knew he had carried out Stephen's wishes in every detail. The committee recognized the surgical skill with which he had cut and pasted the Arlington program into a form more acceptable for FCI management. And all with proper peer review.

Stanley rose slowly. He had waited a long time for this moment. "There is no way to reorient the biotherapy program with Gordon in place. The time has come for him to leave. Just look at these magazines, not to mention the "Today" show. If Phil Donahue is next I think I'll throw up. The man has become a focus of attention, and because of a certain skill he has in dealing with the media coupled with his not inconsequential scientific accomplishments over the past two years, he has become an independent force with which to contend."

"How will you do this?" Fish interrupted, although he knew full well how they would slowly tie the noose around Gordon's neck. He was anxious to get to the point.

"We have begun to turn off the pipeline, and he is already uncomfortable. His personnel actions are moving very slowly. We have halted his request for contract support to expand his laboratory. True, he's been in his new building for about a year, but programs subsequent to that have been sharply truncated. As Sam mentioned, the fermentation program has been cut, and the review process for his protocols has been lengthened. Dr. Gordon is caught in bureaucratic quicksand, and the slowdown is making him quite frustrated. He could wallpaper his office with all the memoranda he's written recently, expressing his dissatisfaction. Instead of buckling down and taking his place in the system, he is, as usual, trying to change the system." People around the table nodded in agreement, so Stanley continued.

"Obviously, this self-preservation attitude can be couched as an individual not working in the best interest of the team, and I have begun to change his Public Health Service work evaluation personnel record in this regard. Slowly, gradually, so it doesn't look like we are ganging up on Mr. Popularity. He is being characterized, on the record, as non-cooperative, not following directives, and combative. Not a team player. In short, we are doing everything we can to make life difficult for him and the program. As a result, his scientists are beginning to feel the crunch. His programs have slowed noticeably." Stanley paused for a sip of water to heighten the drama of the moment.

"I have just finished an internal scientific review of the biotherapy program. It will contain many serious questions with regard to productivity. It will recommend an external scientific peer review (site visit) one year earlier than is usual. Our board of scientific counselors will respond next week with an approval for that external review. It should be completed before the biotherapy program celebrates its third birthday. I'm quite sure that the review committee will find, in a manner similar to our own evaluation, that the program needs more focus and more substance. Dr. Gordon and his illustrious team are in for much anxiety." Stanley was flushed with a deep, curiously sexual excitement as he outlined Robert Gordon's death sentence at the FCI. In addition to serving Stephen, Stanley derived great pleasure in destroying this man. The end of the Gordon problem.

Now it was finally Stephen's turn. All eyes turned to him, but he didn't need to stand, so commanding was his presence. "I'm pleased to receive these reports from Sam and Stanley. Good work. We're on the right track. I, too, have spoken to Dr. Gordon and it is clear that he is feeling a great deal of stress and strain. It's my guess that he will begin to explore possibilities outside of government soon. My own agenda would be for the biotherapy program to be reoriented no later than 1984 and that gives us about a year and a half to complete the process. If we can continue to make life difficult for Robert, and he decides to move his operation elsewhere, that should take him out of the game. He can't possibly produce enough support outside the Arlington program to be a serious contender, and there is no way that he can get sufficient funding through FCI grants and contracts, without our support, to be a competitive force. So we can effectively neutralize him outside the FCI, and then do as we want."

He'd done it again, manipulating the system with words like "reorient" and "focus" to fit his own needs. Over the Musso years, scientist after scientist and program after program had been "restructured", always under the banner of peer review, good science, progress and the public interest. Stephen was a master at the game. A game to which the taxpayer is totally dumb.

"In addition to helping Dr. Gordon see the opportunities outside the FCI, I'd like to outline my general long term plan for biotherapy. It is now apparent to me that genetically-engineered biologicals and monoclonal antibodies will indeed become important players in cancer research and treatment. Monoclonals are proving to be excellent tools in isolating natural substances. Interferon, although not the wonder drug it was touted to be, is at least as good for some cancers as the best chemotherapeutics we have developed so far. The public perception is that it has taken us 30 years to develop 40 toxic drugs, but interferon arrived practically overnight. That doesn't make our drug development efforts look good."

"Now, considering the way things have been progressing, we have to recognize that further interferons, other lymphokines and cytokines, and monoclonal antibodies will be of increasing importance. I am particularly intrigued by conjugated antibodies, getting the little bastards to bring our drugs and radiation to, exactly where they are needed. In light of our very large chemotherapy program, I envision a coalescence of the biotherapy program with our chemotherapy efforts. We must emphasize the view that antibodies are predominantly targeting substances, adjuncts to drugs, and not therapeutic agents on their own. The press must pick this up too."

"This arrangement is the only way to continue to fund drug development at the level we are accustomed to, yet incorporate this increasingly popular new approach as well. It's the best of both worlds. We will have had the insight and foresight to initiate the biotherapy program in 1980, and the creativity to integrate it into existing modalities once it had become established. By 1988, I expect biotherapy to become a support program for the larger clinical oncology program here in Washington, returning the focus and attention where it should be, here. Now, gentlemen, are there any questions?"

As usual, there were none.

CHAPTER 17

THE BREAK

Summer 1983

Robert was sitting, once again, in the corner settee in Dr. Lizzard's office, as Stanley finished his telephone conversation. The phone dropped back into its cradle, and Stanley walked slowly over to the adjacent chair. He gave Robert a sidelong look.

"I suppose you know why I called you in today."

"Not exactly, but I suspect it has to do with a continuation of our previous discussions."

"Yes, I think you need to take some action. Stephen just called me about a letter you sent to the chairman of the board of the Denbow Pharmaceutical Company. Apparently, and correct me if I am wrong, in that letter you suggested the structure for an institute to be funded by the pharmaceutical company. Is that so?"

"Yes, Bill Carothers and I have known each other for years. He has asked me on several occasions to describe a structure in which research in the area of biotherapy might best be conducted. I drew up a plan for a non-profit institute funded by Denbow Pharmaceuticals with the discoveries of the institute accruing to the company for the commercial return. Bill asked me to put that in a form of a proposal and, considering the climate here, I did," Robert replied in his usual up-front manner.

"Stephen says that's a problem. He is very concerned about that communication," Stanley stated, a smirk at the corner of his mouth.

Robert was alert at Stanley's misuse of the word "concern," part of that special FCI language that included "focus," "reorient" and "restructure," terms that on the surface were positive, but really signalled impending doom for someone or some program. When Stephen Musso expressed a "concern," it didn't mean that he cared about something, but that that something, or someone, was impinging on his own territory, and must be stopped.

"To what aspect of this proposal does Stephen have a concern?" Robert asked with a mock innocence that was apparently lost on Stanley.

"Well, at the moment, you are director of the biotherapy program for the FCI, a program which hands out $20 million a year in contracts and grants. And some of this funding goes to pharmaceutical companies to produce various biological substances for us. Now, don't you think you are getting yourself into a conflict of interest situation, and to make matters even more suspicious, at the very same time that you are in a sign-off position with approval power for the Institute? Stephen thinks so."

"At least part of what you say is true. Over the last four years we have indeed supported pharmaceutical companies in the manner you describe. But Denbow Pharmaceuticals has never been on that list, nor are they currently vying for funding. You know well that a contract with us takes more than a year from initial approval to activation. Since Denbow has no such current applications, and we all agree that my time here is limited, I can hardly see how a conflict of interest can arise when no relationship is in place or planned between the FCI and this company."

"Nonetheless," countered Stanley, obviously enjoying this, "there is the potential for conflict of interest and certainly the appearance of it. And this creates a real problem for Stephen."

Stephen and his potential problems, Robert thought, always orchestrated to eliminate some threat. Why was this invented conflict of interest a "problem" when it wasn't considered a problem for Stephen to alter the review process to get rid of George Trumpey? Or to change the committee in the peer review system to re-re-evaluate Dr. Cliner's grant to give it a higher score to appease an outspoken Senator? Why wasn't it a conflict of interest to influence Congress right and left in its granting of funds? More political horse manure, more "problems" and "concerns" and now "conflicts of interest." Robert could hardly keep up with all the fabricated situations.

Why couldn't Stephen and Stanley have the guts to state the obvious, that they had decided that it was time for him to make an official announcement of resignation? This Denbow proposal is just a smokescreen, and they all knew it. Robert decided to steer the conversation more towards the real issues. After all, at this point, what did he have to lose?

"Stanley, we discussed several months ago my interest in leaving the FCI," he began tentatively. Stanley said nothing. "You assured me that there would be no public announcements, since that might interfere with my ability to compete for positions outside the government. In spite of that promise, rumors have circulated to that effect -- and it hasn't been difficult to trace them to your office. So you haven't held up your end of the bargain." And then it came pouring out. "Isn't it bad enough that you twist things, invent things, to speed my departure to suit your own needs? Must you add petty backstabbing to the list?"

Robert stopped for a minute to control his rising anger and frustration, but to his surprise, Stanley denied nothing. So he continued. "Look, I don't want to argue, I know it's useless. I know this Denbow business is just a part of the plan. Tell Stephen he can save his energy and "concern". I am willing to officially resign my position this fall as director if I'm given the opportunity to work for about four more months in Arlington. My current situation involves a new opportunity beginning in February, and I can finish my work here by then," Robert responded.

Finally Stanley spoke. "I don't have any problem with that arrangement. Please make the announcement soon so this matter can be cleared up," he said curtly.

Robert had never been given to violence, but the feelings surging through him at that moment were undeniable. He said nothing, but stood up slowly, towering over the Lizard. Robert stood a little too closely to Lizzard, letting the other man appreciate his physical power, and his suppressed rage. Stanley backed away uncomfortably, leading the way to the door. But Robert wasn't quite finished.

"You know, this is my fourth year back at the FCI at the 'executive level'. I've learned a great deal, particularly from you, Roger and Stephen. It's taken me awhile, but I understand finally how the 'family' works, and how the "in" group arranges its business, and everyone else's, for that matter. One day there'll be an accounting. The purpose of this publicly funded Institute, in case you've forgotten, is to develop new methods to heal the sick. And that's precisely what I've done -- even you can't disparage my scientific record. But you bastards are using it like your own playground, for your own cancer-like egos, to enhance your own scientific and personal reputations. Yes, I'll resign, and it will be effective this fall. But I can tell you this, I'm going to build a system that works better, and I'm going to see that the public understands how people like you abuse them. You can be sure that this story is not over." And he stormed out, slamming the door behind a somewhat surprised Stanley Lizzard.

Stanley's first impulse was to laugh at Robert's characteristic naivetee. But something about that emotion-charged speech got to Stanley. He didn't feel sorry for Robert's dismantled career, he didn't like the man anyway. But Stanley was a little bit uneasy. Sure, they could arrange for him to leave, but Robert Gordon was a very bright man, and one who was extremely popular with the press, who would be all too happy to listen to his tale of woe. Yes, he could be dangerous, even after he leaves. Long after.

Robert was getting worried. He had been in conversations with Bill Carothers and the Denbow Pharmaceutical Company for months. They were interested, in fact very interested, in his proposal to build a non-profit cancer research institute. Unfortunately, they were unable to make the commitment to fund it, at least at the necessary level.

In his proposal, Robert had described a massive effort requiring $5 million per year, and a laboratory/clinical research facility that might occupy 50,000 square feet and employ up to 150 people. This Biotherapy Institute would develop new leads in cancer treatment, leads which would convey commercial possibilities directly to Denbow. He suggested a five year commitment from the company, which amounted to a $25 million arrangement.

It was an unprecedented request in terms of amount and time, Bill Carothers had gently told him.

Bill respected Robert very much. He had known him for many years, knew Robert was a man of action and deed. Given all this, he also knew Denbow Pharmaceuticals, a major firm that had built its success on tranquilizers and antacids. They had a single anticancer drug, and it was not a big money maker. Several antivirals were in development, but these were years away from commercial success. The company's interest in cancer was serious, but fledgling. And although he felt sure that as CEO he could drum up enough support to establish the institute that Robert proposed, he also knew that $1 million per year would be the maximum Denbow support.

Bill and Robert sat on the porch of a modest glass and wood frame house on the coast of North Carolina. It was one of those pleasant fall evenings with the warm breezes flowing across the porch, and the sun setting over the trees behind the house. Bill, Robert and their families had vacationed together in the Carolinas before, but this time, it was just the two of them. Robert needed desperately to get away from Stanley Lizzard and his ominous meetings. He hadn't counted on frustrations with Denbow.

"I'm disappointed, damn disappointed," said Robert. "I'd hoped that Denbow might be the source for support for this institute. I tried to interest Mallory but they were negative."

"As you know, I've come up with good clinical support from the Good Samaritan Hospital near Atlanta," Robert continued. "Mary Margaret and the kids are all prepared for me to be at home for a change, but none of it works without support for the research, nothing works without the Biotherapy Institute."

"I know, I know," answered Bill. "I'm disappointed, too. I've been to my Board on three occasions, and this is the best I can do. If I try to come up with more, it will damage my credibility. Robert, you've been a success in everything you've done and everybody knows it, but this company has never made this kind of commitment to anyone, and it's not about to fund your project at the level you propose. I suggest that you go forward on a smaller scale. Maybe next year or the year after you can make the case for more support, and Denbow might be convinced to bite off a larger chunk," Bill said quietly.

He did feel his friend's pain. He knew that Robert had spent four years trying to make things happen in government. And he had succeeded, at least scientifically. He understood the frustration of having had major resources available and the difficulty of not being able to use them in what Robert considered to be the best interests of his patients. He also could appreciate the difficulty in leaving the prestigious FCI and taking a big step down in terms of level of support. But he just couldn't do more.

"Bill, I'm going for a run. Want to come?" Robert looked close to tears.

"No, you go ahead. I'll just rest here for awhile." He knew Robert needed time alone. Running would help him work through his feelings.

Robert laced up his Nike Airs. He had used many brands, but for the last five years had stayed with Nike. They were straight lattice shoes, and looked like they could fit on either foot, but they were comfortable and didn't give him any foot or knee problems. He tightened the laces and pulled on his red silk running shorts and, shirtless, headed off down the beach.

How he loved to run! The rhythmic pounding was therapeutic. He ran the roads, the golf courses, the shopping centers, the sidewalks. Wherever he traveled he brought his running shoes with him. You never needed a partner for this. You can go any time, any place and release energy and work on frustration.

And he certainly had a lot to work on.

Robert loved the beach best. The sound of the waves, the soft impact on the sand, the people to watch, and the occasional pretty girl all added to the uplifting effect. His feet pounded away, his pace a bit more rapid than usual, the extra exertion showing in his shortness of breath. He felt a vague, unfamiliar discomfort in his upper abdomen. Must be the pizza he'd had for lunch. Slowing down the pace somewhat seemed to help. So he continued his run until he was about five miles out on the North Carolina coast; then turned around and jogged back towards Bill's cabin.

Robert used these runs to bat around the germ of an idea. He now knew that he couldn't work within the political confines of government. There was plenty of money, but too little attention to the patient, too much bureaucracy, too much self-service. The review procedures were ridiculous, even on the rare occasions when they actually worked.

But by the same token, the university system was a dinosaur, steeped in tradition and conservatism to the point that things moved too damn slowly to get any quality research accomplished. The universities with which he had been associated were all the same. Unending questions. "What impact will your work have on the department of biochemistry? On the department of physiology? Has the dean approved it? Why are you moving so fast?" Like the government, the university was rigid and institutionalized, with the added problem of lack of funding. They offered big packages, yet when you arrived, graduate students and post-docs in tow, commitments began to melt away. Subtle and not-so-subtle pressures to spend more and more time writing grant proposals became a way of life. Within a year or two, the package began to look far less attractive, and the investigator found himself looking for greener pastures. So the national research picture was a stream of researchers moving from place to place in vain search of the perfect setting, the university or government institution with funds, but without bureaucracy.

Robert was beginning to think that the atmosphere to do the type of research that should be done just didn't exist.

What then of the pharmaceutical industry? The companies were large, had lots of cash and understood the value of research and development. It was on a 12 mile that Robert had first come up with this possibility. And although it seemed a viable option, biotherapy was not a typical research endeavor. It required enormous amounts of money, and precious time. He had thought that Denbow would be the answer, but even they couldn't provide the necessary level of funding to develop the critical mass needed to carry out his programs. Well, thought Robert as his pace slowed to seven minutes a mile, I could go around to various other companies. But none are as flexible or financially sound as Denbow, and in none of them do I have a friend like Bill Carothers.

But Robert wasn't out of ideas. His pace unconsciously rose to 6:30 a mile as he once again went through the details. Privatization.

It was a word that he kept seeing in the newspaper and hearing on the news. The current Republican administration was popularizing the concept that certain things could be done better by private industry than by government. Maybe the principles of privatization could be applied to research.

Could research be privatized? Certainly pharmaceutical companies did research, and that was in the private sector. Most pharmaceutical companies were considered to have rather staid research departments, and high quality university scientists tended to look down their noses at them. Even at meetings there was a clear delineation between the "academic" investigators and those who lowered themselves to work for the corporate sector.

But things were changing. At first the academic people had turned up their collective noses at the new tiny companies sprouting up on the west coast like some new type of crop -- first Genentech, then Cetus, now Conjugation Technology. Gradually the ambiance was changing, and the scientific staffs of these aggressive start-ups became peppered with some of the most respected names in university science. Now the academic and pharmaceutical groups at meetings were beginning to be bridged by the fledgling field of biotechnology. In fact, communications were rocketing back and forth between the various groups in an unprecedented fashion. A change was clearly in the air and Robert intended to at least learn from it, if not become a part of it.

"Maybe, just maybe, I can do what I want to do privately," he thought aloud as he neared the cabin. However, there was still the question of money. Private companies got money from investors, right? But that meant profits. The entity would have to be set up as a for-profit company to generate the needed investor interest.

But that would never work. A for-profit cancer research facility? Everybody and his brother would be taking pot-shots at it. And him. He could imagine the headlines, "getting rich off the sick", "Separating terminal cancer patients from their money", "cash for cures". It would be a circus. He'd be compared to Lawrence of Arabia, that quack zoologist in the Caribbean who runs a bogus cancer treatment center. No, there has to be some other way.

The cabin was in sight, and his pace was up to 6 minutes. This was when his heart really began pounding, when he felt 10 years younger, 12 pounds lighter and 2 minutes faster. He could hear the crowd scream. He could see the ball sailing toward the basket. He could feel the lift that came with the swish. The memories fluttered through his endorphin-soaked brain as he finished his 10 miles.

Exhausted, drenched, he did his usual 10 minute walk to allow his heart rate to come down slowly, a strategy that reduced the risk of post-exercise heart irregularity. As he walked by the cabin, he looked up at Bill, asleep with his feet propped up on the porch. He's a good man, and he's in the private sector, Robert thought. His company operates ethically and they make a profit. In fact, hadn't their brightly colored annual report stated that their 1982 before tax margin for drugs for the sick and terminally ill was about 26%?

And doctors in private practice -- weren't they "profiting" from the sick? In medical personal corporations, doctors didn't sell stock, but they were really the shareholders. Wasn't that medicine for a profit? Hospitals, both for profit and non profit, delivered care for a fee. And what about universities? He thought back to some of the institutions with which he had been affiliated, remembering particularly the dean at Mallory. He was always so interested in "bottom line," as he like to say. At meetings the dean had stressed over and over that Mallory could only function if revenues exceeded expenses, using the term "net fund balance." He'd used that phrase in the same sentence as "non-profit" and "philanthropic." So no matter how institutions defined themselves, money was, and would always be, important. Only the government could operate with expenses higher than revenue.

Robert turned to walk back towards the cabin. Was there really any difference between a net fund balance and a profit? Didn't profits go to the investors in the form of dividends? Didn't net fund balances get used to support the constituencies of Mallory? He recalled the office building next to Mallory Hospital, constructed with net fund balance dollars. It was 12 stories of glass and steel, on a par with the finest corporate office facilities in the country. Well appointed in finish and furnishings, the physicians' offices looked like they came from a magazine spread. The conference rooms were deeply carpeted, with tables of solid walnut and moldings of solid handcut cherry. The athletic club in the basement was top notch, as was the private dining room. All from the net fund balance.

But the examining rooms were extraordinarily plain. And the patient waiting rooms bordered on shabby. Don't let the patient understand that surplus funds exist!

The doctors were the constituency for the university. If they didn't put their patients in Mallory Hospital, then those revenues couldn't exceed expenses. Net fund balances to reward physicians; was it any different than making a profit for an investor?

Forgetting his exhaustion, Robert bounded up the stairs, past Bill who was snoring gently in the rocking chair, his pipe a distant memory on the floor. Soaked with sweat, his ideas coming rapid fire one after the other, Robert grabbed his dictaphone and began to speak as he walked back out to the beach. He quickly sketched out the structure of the company he envisioned. His Biotherapy Institute could easily be folded into this paradigm. If he couldn't get Denbow to fund his concept, he would create a company that would! He added investors and capital, thought about the annual report, and the bottom line.

What Dr. Robert Gordon hastily, but thoughtfully, drew up on that beautiful North Carolina fall afternoon was a crude business plan, one that would bring research directly to the patient, privatizing a process that had been a government/university/pharmaceutical company monopoly for more than half a century.

He had conceived of a process that might well revolutionize developmental therapeutics and the very practice of medicine. Cancer Therapeutics Incorporated was born!

CHAPTER 18

CANCER THERAPEUTICS INC.

January 1984

Whoever invented the concept of hell obviously wasn't familiar with New York City in the midst of a January blizzard. The wind was howling off the East river, blending the fishy, garbage odor of the river with the stench pouring from the decaying factories upstream. Snow blew relentlessly out of the northeast on the frigid wind. It was a day to match the coldness of the New York City heart.

This was not a city for which Robert had great affinity. Compared to the infectious warmth of the southerners to which he was accustomed, the truly "ugly" New Yorker was rude, hurried, and often downright nasty. Fights were commonplace in the filthy streets, where drunks and whores mingled like flotsam bobbing in the East River. Sometimes for amusement he'd turn on the evening news -- murder after murder, and people weren't the least bit shocked. In his hometown, one murder a year was considered a major crime wave.

Maybe if you had a fancy Park Avenue apartment and a limousine, life in the Rotten Apple might be tolerable. The cabbies drove Robert particularly crazy, with their incessant honking and shouting. But once when he had complained, a colleague had commented that the subway was far worse than any cab ride, and dared him to ride the "D" train. Robert had accepted the dare, and as he had descended the stairs into the station had felt as if he were entering a giant toilet, so overpowering was the reek of urine. So he put up with the cabs.

He and Thomas Hastings had managed to survive this cab ride, and were now making their way in the blinding snow to a rather dilapidated building on Wall Street. They were pushed through the massive doors by a crowd of people, past a dingy newsstand and before they had a chance to check the address, found themselves being packed into an elevator.

"Tom, are you sure this is it?" asked Robert as he glanced at a fat woman reading an X-rated magazine hidden behind a U.S. News and World Report at the shabby newsstand. "Looks kind of seedy to me."

"Don't be deceived by outward appearances," answered Tom as the elevator doors closed, packing the people in like so many sardines. "This is indeed the place. And the Wall Street firm of Berle, Eintoven and Toban has provided venture capital to some of the best known companies in the country. Berle, Eintoven and Toban. What an unholy alliance it is."

"What do you mean?" Robert asked. Tom seemed unusually sensitive to people's ethnic origins.

"An Englishman, a German, and a Polish Jew. Wonder how they got together, and what makes their chemistry work?" Tom said, more to himself than to Robert, who couldn't hear above the annoying Muzak anyway.

Tom's interest in origins stemmed from the fact that he considered himself to be a hybrid, his father a WASP and his mother a Jew. He had always felt that he had the best of both worlds -- the regal appearance and demeanor of his father, his shrewd intelligence and quest for knowledge from his mother. Tom had majored in philosophy as an undergraduate, then headed straight for his M.B.A. at Wharton, where he graduated with honors. But he had realized that an M.B.A. without some other sort of expertise was not enough, so he had begun studying all sorts of subjects, finally concentrating on molecular biology, which was gradually evolving into biotechnology. And today, he was Vice President of a small biotech company in Seattle, but interested in moving into a larger operation.

When the door opened on the 12th floor, Robert immediately thought of Dorothy opening the door of her creaky old house and looking out in amazement at the stunning beauty of the Land of Oz.

Berle, Eintoven and Toban, whatever their origins, had obviously made a dollar or two from their investments. The area onto which the elevator opened was not gaudy, but expensively decorated with two enormous leather armchairs at either end of a glass table displaying a nice selection of classy magazines -- Business Week, Harper's, the Atlantic Monthly. Some contrast to the sleazy fare he had glimpsed downstairs, Robert thought. They entered the double glass doors, and were greeted by a rather out-of-place looking receptionist.

"May I help you?" Frazzled black hair, a beakish nose and full red lips with a rather used look. Not at all like the well-kept, attractive young GS-10s flitting about government, Robert mused. But despite her rather frowzy appearance, she was pleasant and efficient, not to mention unusually polite for a resident of this baffling city.

"Yes," Tom responded. "My name is Tom Hastings, and this is Dr. Robert Gordon. We're here to see Mr. Toban."

"Oh, we've been expecting you. Please come with me." Robert noticed when she stood that she had a spectacular figure. Actually, all she needed was a nose job and a hairdresser; then she wouldn't be all that bad. He realized his mind was wandering because he was a bit nervous.

Tom and Robert followed her into a large and heavily decorated conference room. The walls were lined with plaques and awards, signifying successful public offerings, bonds, conversions, and a variety of other business initiatives the firm had accomplished. A bar stretched halfway across one wall, filled with a wide variety of beverages, and a young woman scuttled back and forth carrying hors d'ouvres. At the far end was a black leather couch and a telephone. Filling the middle of the enormous room was a gigantic, solid walnut conference table surrounded by beautiful highback leather chairs, with what looked like room to seat a small army. The far wall was all glass and looked out over the bustling Wall Street community. Tom tried to squeeze his 6'4" frame into a small closet to hand up their coats.

Robert looked at his colleague and thought that the man could benefit from an exercise program. At 40, he was nearing an age when last night's dinner seemed to hang around the jowls and belt line. He still looked fairly athletic, but Robert could tell that without some work it would soon be lost. His mind was wandering again.

Tom Hastings had first approached Robert at the FCI, trying to convince him to buy interferon from his Seattle firm. He had gone through all the calculations to show how their blood bank source and a special extraction method could produce interferon less expensively than the competition. And Robert had blown him out of the water with his ensuing lecture on the benefits of genetically engineering interferon.

Hastings was hooked. This recombinant DNA stuff was better in every conceivable way -- cheaper, purer, more plentiful. It was Robert who had initially alerted Tom to the economic opportunities afforded by this new wave of applied molecular biology.

When Robert had shown his embryonic business plan to Bill Carothers on that important fall day, Bill agreed that it was an arrangement that might work, but he added that it would need a brilliant person with a keen business sense and a thorough understanding of the scientific principles to get it off the ground. And if it could be launched, then Denbow might be interested -- very interested -- in pitching in.

Bill Carothers had someone in mind. A sharp young guy he had tried to hire about a year earlier, and saw infrequently at meetings. His name was Tom Hastings. He had turned down Bill's offer because he didn't want to become part of a large company -- he wanted to build one. Robert remembered his own positive impressions of Hastings, and so had contacted him.

And so the partnership with Tom was the first of several strokes of good fortune for Cancer Therapeutics Inc., the name that Tom and Robert had agreed upon. CTI was conceived to serve the cancer patient directly with biological-based therapeutics. Incorporating the practice of medicine and research capability within the firm provided a direct line of delivery from the laboratory to the patient. Robert, Tom and Bill, when they had finally gotten together to discuss the project, were enthusiastic that the concept could work.

The massive door opened, and a portly gentleman of perhaps 60 entered. His hand was outstretched as he waddled slightly coming forward. "I'm Richard Toban."

"Robert Gordon, and this is Tom Hastings," Robert responded.

"Gentlemen, would you like something to drink before we talk about your company? Diet cola is all I'm allowed, but we have a little white wine, if you'd like," he offered.

"Just decaffeinated coffee for us," Robert said.

After the introduction of two junior staffers working with Mr. Toban, they all sat at one end of the massive conference table.

"Well, I've had a chance to look over your business plan for Cancer Therapeutics. There are some things about it I like and some that trouble me. Perhaps we could discuss your concept for a few minutes," he began, then paused to sip his Diet Coke. Although Richard Toban was heavy, Robert could see the residual of a powerful athletic frame. He like the direct eye contact and the firm handshake of the man. The pause gave Robert a few seconds to wonder whether his concern would be business or science related. It turned out to be neither.

"I'm worried about the ethics involved. Won't there be a problem with patients paying for experimental treatment?"

Robert was ready. "Well, this company is structured to allow the patient to fund research in his own behalf, and that research may indeed beget a treatment for that patient. It is a research service company, designed to use current laboratory techniques for the benefit of the patient. We're not really a product-oriented company like a pharmaceutical house. We sell research and support services, not products," said Robert.

"But patients paying for research, isn't that going to be difficult? Seems to me that research is presently funded by the Federal Cancer Institute, the American Cancer Society and the United Way. Will people really pay for research?" asked Toban.

"Well, I think they will pay for opportunity, which is what we're really offering here," Robert continued. "The research laboratory now has the power to make certain biological substances for use in treatment. We can, for example, make genetically-engineered lymphokines. We can develop growth and maturation factors, and we can surely make monoclonal antibodies. Each of these has a potential role in cancer treatment, and each can be applied eventually to potentially benefit the patient funding the research. I think it is a scenario that an intelligent patient can understand," Robert said with enthusiasm. They had commissioned a patient acceptance study and it confirmed Robert's own sense from ministering to cancer patients. Patients wanted more access to research-based experimental treatment and, if able, would pay for it. He and Tom had been through all of these potential problems quite thoroughly, even testing each other on how they would respond when asked. And they had decided to be as open and direct as possible.

"Okay, I can see that. Yes, patients might pay for research if they really think it might help them, if they can live long enough for treatment to be developed. But what about guarantees? Will everyone contracting research receive treatment? And if so, will it work? What will happen when it doesn't?" said Mr. Toban.

"Well, that is a problem. It's true that the research will not be fruitful every time -- research never is, and doesn't come with guarantees. Patients will sign up for the service under a research contract agreement and there will be a strong element of disclosure and informed consent. Yes, it's possible that the patients, particularly those unfamiliar with scientific research, will be unable to understand the percentages involved, the fact that what they're paying for may not work, and that at present we cannot predict with 100% accuracy when it will and when it won't. And I'm sure we will become the focus of attention when our business plan becomes known, because it is so novel. But I'm absolutely convinced that what we offer is something that many cancer patients and their families will welcome," Robert said, rather passionately.

"What exactly do you mean?" asked Mr. Toban.

"I've taken care of cancer patients for the past 15 years and it is my view that they want more control in the process. To be told nothing can be done is devastating to the patient and the family. Even an effort that is not ultimately successful may have some benefit in that at least the patient and the family feel that they are doing everything possible to directly fight the disease."

"But can't patients for whom conventional therapy does not work just sign up for a government sponsored trial for experimental therapy?"

"It's not that simple, not for most people. Our current system rejects so many people, so many more than are actually selected for treatment. The patient is too tall, too short, too fat, too thin, too green, too blue! In some protocols unless you're an Olympic athlete with a tiny nodule in your lung, you're simply ineligible for that treatment. And, the more promising the approach, like these new biotherapies, the more restrictive the entry criteria."

"I don't follow. Wouldn't a government-supported trial want to include as many different types of people as possible?" Toban asked.

"You must remember that government and university programs are designed primarily to write papers and answer science questions. Their focus is the experimental protocol and maximizing the chance of a positive study. This leads to a medical journal paper and more government funding for their system. Patient care is really secondary. Their primary interest is in taking the best shot. So, to get results, they only enter patients who are most likely to respond to the treatment. I don't have to tell you that this excludes many, many patients who might benefit from experimental treatment. It's a fact that the public doesn't understand well, but believe me, I've lived it during my past four years at the FCI."

Much relieved to have gotten this across to an obviously fascinated listener, Robert now sat back, and outlined exactly how the research contract worked and how the company might perform research for patients.

Of course, much of the "company" still existed only in Robert's head. What he had at that moment was a few sheets of paper, Tom Hastings, a major shareholder in Denbow, and a number of private investors willing to invest in the concept. What they needed now was a lead venture capitalist, a company with a strong reputation in the investment banking world who could get their company well capitalized and eventually take them public with a large stock offering.

"Let's get back to the ethics. You're putting yourself in a tenuous position, don't you think, Dr. Gordon? You're going to take these desperate peoples' money, do research for them, develop some exotic treatments, and then actually treat the patients yourself. That's not the way medicine is usually done. A for-profit company inventing, developing and treating the patient all in one fell swoop. A situation in which the conflict of interest issue and your motivations are likely to be questioned. That sounds pretty radical. Wait til Phil Donahue gets wind of it!" With that, Mr. Toban leaned back and smiled. He had already bought the concept himself, but he wanted to see how this young physician handled these disturbing sorts of questions. He knew they would arise again and again.

Richard Toban was well aware of the truth in all that Dr. Gordon said. Too well aware, for he had watched for three years as his brother had died of colon cancer which had spread to the liver. Each year there had been more pain, further weight loss, and more interference with daily activities. Until the end, his brother had struggled to go to work and to try to maintain some semblance of normal life. And throughout that time, he and the family had searched frantically throughout the world for an opportunity just like Dr. Gordon was outlining.

Toban's brother had been 67 at the time of his illness, just a few years older than Toban himself now was. Too old for a promising FCI study of chemotherapy to the liver. Too fragile for a Sloan-Kettering study of a substance to make the body manufacture its own interferon. Too sick for M.D. Anderson, where the initial interferon trials were being done. Toban wished that Robert Gordon and his wild new plan had been around when Philip was ill. He would have been the first to sign up -- and he suspected that there would be no shortage of customers, once the inevitable media hoopla died down.

Throughout Richard Toban's reverie, Robert had been defending his concept, and was now concluding his argument forcefully. "Let's use the resources of the individual to begin to make the machinery work. Let's 'prime the pump' with private investor funding for the individual and see if that can't make things happen. Let's allow privatization the opportunity to succeed." Robert slumped back in his chair, exhausted.

Richard Toban was a capitalist. He had invested in many, many opportunities, most of which had prospered. So he knew what it took to make a business go -- a man with foresight and a better mousetrap and a willing and able market. All of these elements were here for CTI, and he was indeed interested. His penetrating gaze moved now to Tom Hastings, who had been rather quiet so far.

"Mr. Hastings, do you have anything to add?"

"Yes, sir, I do think this can be a sound business. I'm sure you have looked over the financial projections and you can see that our strategy is to begin this operation with very narrow margins and very little bricks and mortar. Once we're able to prove the concept works -- and I have little doubt that it will -- we then intend to build a company with regional offices and satellite joint ventures with physicians and hospitals to offer our services across the country. Eventually we see a network circling the globe. I think Robert has the science right, and I believe that I can make the business work."

Mr. Toban stood up and paced one time around the gargantuan table as if doing laps. He then looked out the broad expanse of glass on the east wall. He turned slowly from the window and looked back at the two men.

"There's no way that this firm can support your business. It will be too controversial, it's too new, it's too avant-garde, and it looks too chancy. I'm disappointed to tell you this since I personally feel a strong sense of confidence in both the business and the science. However, Berle, Eintoven and Toban have prospered by taking early phase but well understood concepts to obvious markets and doing that more efficiently than the others. There is simply too much uncertainty here for our firm to become involved."

The disappointment was evident on both Robert and Tom's faces, who looked like they had each lost a brother. The weight of this trip to New York City was now bearing down on Robert. First, at Bill Carothers' suggestions, they had visited six firms in Boston, and now they had come to here. This was the eighth firm in New York with whom they had held discussions. They would come into the room and present the concept to the company with slides, both Robert and Tom participating on cue in the carefully-crafted presentation, a so-called "dog and pony show." At the conclusion, they would answer questions. Ethics? Patients paying for research? Success rates? What will the FCI think? What about the FDA? Shouldn't this be done at a university? Is it a business? Although there had been a few nibbles of interest, neither Tom nor Robert felt that a strong commitment was forthcoming from the previous 14 firms. A leader was needed. These firms might invest if a lead venture capitalist validated the concept with a check. So their hope hadn't diminished because Bill had told them that Mr. Toban was their best bet. If anyone on Wall Street would support their concept, it would be Richard Toban.

Well, here they were. Only a brief series of questions and a rejection. Tom stood and Robert shortly followed.

"We're sorry your firm won't be able to participate. We had looked forward to your leadership. Capital from Berle, Eintoven and Toban would have been the final link in the chain," Tom responded. Poor Dr. Gordon looked too stricken to speak, Toban thought sympathetically.

"Relax, sit a moment." An easy smile fluttered onto Toban's face. "The company won't go for the deal, but I'm personally interested. And I think I know a better way to go about making this a business. Let me sketch out what I have in mind."

As Robert and Tom looked at each other in suppressed jubilation, Mr. Toban walked over the a white board adjacent to the conference table and took out one of the colored pens. "I see this as a multi-staged financing with two initial steps. As I understand it, you have Denbow Pharmaceuticals in for 10% and a series of private investors willing to take 40%. I will personally commit to putting up the other 50% of the capital needed to initiate CTI. Based on your own plans, my investment should total about $5 million. That, plus the other sources, should give you sufficient cash to run for nearly two years. If the patient revenues turn out to be as projected, your cash position should never fall below $3 million during that two year period."

Toban paused to look down at Tom and Robert, but they seemed to be in shock, so he continued. "It is my view that a public offering would be appropriate sometime between year one and year two, depending upon your level of progress. When the time for the public offering comes, I know the mechanism to carry it off."

"Go on," Robert prompted in an uncharacteristically squeaky voice.

"The way I see it, one of two possibilities exists. Hopefully, you will have become more real and accepted, and the questions I brought up a few minutes ago will have been answered or at least satisfactorily approached. If so, this firm will surely be interested in an investment banking relationship to take you public in 1985 or 1986. On the other hand, if my confidence continues but CTI doesn't develop as quickly as we expect, I have a relationship with several smaller investment banking houses which may be interested in a public offering. Either way, I think we can work together to create sufficient capital to get this company up and running."

He walked away from the board where he had been outlining his plan, and over to the two men. He put out his hand. "Gentlemen, I have a very important appointment to keep in Midtown and the car is waiting. If I am late for the reception my wife has planned, we are all in trouble. I will leave you with my two associates to work out the details. Let's get this business rolling."

With a broad smile, he shook Tom's hand. Tom was in a daze. He had hoped that the company might take 20% of the stock and be a lead venture capital banker in the deal. Their lead would then get others interested, and the stock could be sold privately, with a lot of work and a series of further dog and pony shows. But never in his wildest dreams did he expect Mr. Toban to come forward personally and complete the financial arrangement in one meeting.

Robert too appeared to be in shock, but to him the commitment seemed less bizarre. From the beginning, he had had the sense that Richard Toban was a man of special insight. It wasn't anything he had said or done, nothing that Robert could put his finger on, but his presence in the room, his direct stare and the intensity of his interest conveyed a sense of confidence in the concept of CTI. The questions seemed merely to test the waters to see if the men were of tough enough stuff to carry the dream through. He had liked and respected Mr. Toban instantly, despite his devil's advocate play.

"Thank you, sir, both Tom and I are looking forward to a long and positive relationship. The confidence you have shown in us is most gratifying. We will work very hard to justify your decision."

"I'm sure you will, Dr. Gordon, and Tom, I'm sure you will conduct the business in fine fashion. Tom, I'd like you to give me a call next week. I've got some suggestions on potential staff for the business side and some contacts here in New York you may find helpful. Just give me a call on my private line."

With that Mr. Toban handed Tom a plain white business card and left the room. Tom and Robert sat across the table from Mr. Toban's junior counterparts. Paper moved back and forth. A formal written proposal had already been prepared, and Tom was scrutinizing it. Meanwhile, Toban's associates made notes on some background material Tom had provided.

As was often the case, Robert's attention wandered as the business details were being worked out. What a relief this meeting had been! In the other firms they had consulted, the final pronouncement was always the same; "If you increase the price of the research contract, you can increase the profit margins. We'd be very interested in this deal if you could just get the margins up."

But he and Tom had decided from the very beginning not to increase the margins. They felt the margins were reasonable for the patient and the investor. Robert would find patients who felt that making a profit while carrying out services in their behalf was reasonable, and Tom would find investors who could also accept reasonable margins. Tom, Robert, Bill and the initial private investors were all in agreement on this. Now, with Mr. Toban's endorsement, the arrangement was sealed.

Cancer Therapeutics was a reality.

Robert was now looking forward to the trip home. One more month at the FCI and then it was back to Atlanta. The strategy was all sketched out in CTI's business plan, but it was also indelibly inked in Robert's frontal lobe. He was going to demonstrate that the privatization of research could result in benefit for the patient and society. He was going to demonstrate that the government/academic system actually contained margins far greater than a private system. And the margins included dollars that "took care of" the multiple constituencies in the system and, in addition, contained the nonmonetary margins of the system, an academic currency to reward by higher title, greater venue and more power. He was going to demonstrate that a for-profit firm could service patients and deliver technology at a lower cost than the government/academic system, and he was going to demonstrate that all this could be done faster and more efficiently in the private sector.

And he knew what it would take. Capital. Top quality scientists, dedicated technicians, modern laboratory facilities, a good hospital staff, and physicians interested in helping patients. He had always loved assembling teams, and this one would be the best ever! The keynote of the organization would be "service," and the strategy was to develop a company that was patient-centered. They would do research, they would write, they would publish, and they would treat. They would write no laborious grants and would seek no government support. They would do all the things that Robert and his team had done at the FCI before the Musso squeeze, but they would do it in the private sector with the patient's interest first.

That was his commitment.

CHAPTER 19

THE HEADLINE WAS DRAMATIC

Fall 1984

"FCI DIRECTOR DISCOVERS CANCER CAUSED BY VIRUS"

Big damn deal, thought Lydia Green as she tossed the Atlanta Constitution with its enormous headline onto the night table beside her hospital bed. Some good it'll do me.

Lydia Green was a very sick woman. Her painfully enlarged lymph nodes were pushing on her esophagus, causing pain in her chest and an alarming difficulty in swallowing. Engorged abdominal nodes made her look six months pregnant. She had responded to the chemotherapy Dr. Gordon had begun six months ago, but only briefly. But she was used to that, as well as to the nausea, vomiting, low blood counts, every part of her responding, it seemed, except those damn lymphoma cells. At least she didn't lose her hair this time. Her nodes had shrunk a little, but here she was, back in the hospital, still sick, and worst of all, still with no hope for the future.

Distractedly, she picked up the newspaper again and read the tale of how some hot shot, who couldn't even begin to fathom what lymphoma actually felt like, had found some bug he thought caused it.

"Dr. Stephen Musso, director of the prestigious Federal Cancer Institute, announced today the discovery of a virus as the cause of lymphoma, a form of cancer," the article began. Musso's team, included two fellows named Fish and Salla, had made their stellar announcement at a news conference held simultaneously with the publication of their results in the prestigious Journal of Science.

Dr. Musso was asked to describe the importance of the discovery. Maybe, just maybe, thought Lydia, this time it might mean something to me. She read on for the great doctor's response.

> *"This discovery will have long term implications for treatment of patients with lymphoma. We published a preliminary observation of this virus in lymphoma cells in 1982. It has taken us two years of concentrated effort to completely isolate this virus, which we have named human lymphoma/leukemia virus one (HLV-1). The virus can now be produced in our fermentation plant in sufficient quantities to construct a vaccine. Although today we still must use chemotherapy drugs for treatment, the discovery of this virus opens up the opportunity for an anti-viral drug approach in treatment of lymphoma and perhaps, one day, even a vaccine for its prevention. Dr. Salla was the first to describe the class of Herpes virus (HV-A and B) which caused certain non-malignant growths in the mouth, and this same illustrious team isolated HLV-1, the virus which causes lymphoma. I must say, I'm proud of our team effort. Only through the support of public money and the commitment to science above all else has this discovery been possible. I'm pleased to be associated with such a team of dedicated scientists, and I'm gratified to see the public interest and the federal commitment to research translate into a discovery with direct application to patients."*

Lydia was still looking for that missing part about helping patients. Helping one today. The story went on to describe the years of arduous research behind the present shining moment, the efforts of Dr. Salla and his co-workers in the laboratory, and the investigations of Dr. Musso at the FCI in Washington. It recapped Dr. Musso's development of the ABC regimen and checked off many of his accomplishments in the drug treatment of lymphoma and other cancers. Public funding for research and the dedication of the FCI to better treatment was repeatedly emphasized.

Whoopee!, thought Lydia as she lay back in her bed. Dear Abby had more useful information for her than this purported breakthrough did. Great, another discovery she thought. But how does it help me? I'm still in the same nauseatingly green hospital room, taking the same rotten drugs, still sick, sick, sick, she muttered to herself.

Dr. Gordon entered the room to find his normally pleasant patient babbling to herself, fidgeting with the morning's paper. "Hello, Lydia. How are you feeling today?" he asked as he gently touched her shoulder.

"Terrible. I've been sick all night, and I can't swallow any solid foods."

"Well, that's because your lymph nodes are still enlarged. But I think the new chemotherapy is beginning to work. What I wanted to talk to you about, though, is an insurance policy."

"What do you mean, insurance? Is there a problem? I have medical insurance, disability and life insurance, everything, I think," she answered edgily. Why on earth was he bothering a dying woman about insurance? I want to know if the chemotherapy is going to work, and if not, then what? And he talks about insurance, she thought. Dr. Gordon looked strangely excited.

"I'd like to begin a research project with you." He drew up a chair and sat down at her bedside, and she straightened up. She'd long since stopped being nervous about looking so awful in front of such a handsome doctor, but she did subconsciously try to compose herself.

"Well, you asked once why can't we use the body's response to work on your lymphoma. I didn't answer you at the time, but that's exactly what we're trying to do. I've recently been successful in initiating a new enterprise here in Fairfield, and I'd like to ask you to participate in an experiment with me."

"What do you mean by experiment? And what has it got to do with insurance? And my treatment?"

"I'd like to remove one of your enlarged lymph nodes for our laboratory. We'll try to use lymph cells to make an antibody. As you probably realize, judging from the stack of reading material in the corner, we can make antibodies to fight cancer, yours specifically."

"Is it an antibody to this virus that I've been reading about in the paper?" she asked as she handed the paper to Dr. Gordon, who was all too familiar with the FCI tale of glory.

"No, this virus is an important discovery, and it may lead to future treatment, but no, it won't help you today."

Robert scanned the article, marveling once again at the FCI orchestration of this major media event. Pure Musso. They get the research done, or rather their underlings do, then they send the paper to a prestigious journal, and then just before its publication, the FCI propaganda machine, "Cancer Communications," calls all of the major news services and makes a public announcement. If we were to do the same thing in private industry, Robert thought, the FCI would roundly criticize us for hyping the discovery to sell stock. But what are hyping discoveries to increase congressional funding?

"They will get thousands of calls a day in the next few days about his announcement, Lydia. Unfortunately, many patients do not realize, as you do, that it takes many years for a discovery to filter down to practicality." He hated the look of despondency on her face. Giving up would be the very worst thing she could do -- and that was why he was here. "But that's not what I'm here about. When I said insurance, I meant that we can develop some of these antibodies that may stick to your lymphoma cells. If they do, we can hook a drug to the antibody and maybe kill the cancer cells -- and only the cancer cells. Perhaps without vomiting, hair loss and bone marrow damage."

"Where does the insurance come in? Are you speaking figuratively?" Lydia asked, her interest and animation returning.

"In a way. It takes us some time to make the antibodies, but it may represent insurance in the sense of a future experimental treatment being available if we start today. I think these drugs are working, but they may not work next month or next year. Despite how awful you feel, you are otherwise in good shape. I believe this research project might supply you with some insurance, a future experimental option, a definite hope," he explained.

Lydia thought a moment. Something was clearly bothering her. "But what about cost? I've been reading about your 'private' approach. You certainly have become controversial. The newspapers say that you make these antibodies for $50,000 a piece," she answered solemnly. "You know I can't afford that," she added in a low voice.

"Yes, I realize that. Much of our work is indeed expensive, and we've asked patients to fund their own research. But what I'm proposing to you is to have the company fund research for you. For a few patients, medically qualified but financially unable, we're able to do these research projects on a limited basis with research and development monies from CTI. We don't announce this to the newspapers although it would certainly make us look better, because we don't want to get peoples' hopes up and then have to crash them down for lack of money, space and facilities. But, Lydia, you have been my patient for nearly a year now, and I feel I know you and your disease well. You are an excellent candidate. Your medical and mental condition are crucial to the success of our experimental treatment. I have discussed your case with our research committee, and they've agreed to pay the full research contract costs to develop the antibodies for you. Would you like to proceed?"

The relief flooding through Lydia Green was quite apparent. He had tried to get her into a free FCI program but the "slots" were full. Besides, she was sick. Not a great candidate. She began to sob softly and felt an inner joy. Of course she would participate, and she would have reached out to hug Dr. Gordon if only her arms didn't hurt so much. She had been reading and reading and knew all about idiotypes and epitopes and realized that her type of cancer was one that the new biological treatments would be pioneered on. But she hadn't really imagined that she would live long enough to be a "guinea pig" for such a treatment. But this she would gladly do -- she knew the chemotherapy was a stop-gap measure, and she also knew that the FCI virus work meant nothing for her. Dr. Gordon was not offering a guarantee of anything, but he did offer hope. And she realized how important that was.

"Yes, I'd like to participate. I can help myself, and possibly others from what you learn on me. And doctor, I know a great deal more about this than you might think of a poor shopkeeper. I know about the man on the west coast who was treated three years ago with monoclonal antibody and appears to have been cured. These antibodies do indeed look promising, and far less fearful than the drugs I've been getting. I firmly believe that you're on the right track and if I could help and be helped at the same time, that would be terrific." She wondered if he would mind if she hugged him.

Unable to help herself, Lydia burst into tears. It was as if the long years of suffering with her on-again-off-again disease had suddenly become too much to bear. What little family she had had been supportive, but these last few years she had felt so alone. Reading about the immune system and biotherapy had been therapeutic in taking her mind off of her plight, and now she might actually benefit from it. She would gladly sign any forms, give any tissue, come down to the lab herself and climb into a test tube if she had to. And for the first time in her life, she realized, she had complete faith in her physician.

"Okay Lydia. We'll schedule your lymph node biopsy for tomorrow. This process of making antibodies is slow and technically difficult. We need to make several types, so that we can keep ahead of the cancer, attacking whatever sorts of cells might arise from it. I will attempt to link the antibody 'cocktail' to a drug, and we can base that choice on how you've already responded to chemotherapy. And we'll try to get that antibody and its drug cargo to your lymphoma cells, and not your hair, your stomach, or your bone marrow. I'll have my research nurse come around a little later and go over some more details. There is a great deal of paperwork to sign. Let's get going!"

And with that the energetic Dr. Gordon shook his patient's hand and left.

Lydia lay back on the pillow and dropped the newspaper, watching as Stephen Musso's face soaked up a small puddle of green fluid on the floor that had dripped from a hanging plant. For the first time in weeks, Lydia noticed the trees outside her window, was aware of the smallness of the room. She suddenly felt alive again. Her search for a cure was finally showing progress. She would beat this thing, she really would. Between her confidence and dedication, Dr. Gordon's brilliance and her own body's immunological arsenal, they'd do it.

She felt in her innermost being that this was the best approach, the only approach left, for her.

CHAPTER 20

THE CASE

Spring 1985

Daniel Weil fidgeted, squirmed, jerked and rolled around in his bed. He had been sick all night with a growing pressure and sense of fullness in the left part of his chest that he didn't like one bit. He knew the tumor was growing, could actually feel it. He knew he was in trouble.

He also knew he had pushed the system to the limit, to no avail. It had actually been easy getting into the interferon trial. All he'd had to do was make a few calls to the right people. He was well acquainted with pushing political buttons, particularly as it pertained to his cancer. He had Musso, Fish and Lizzard under his thumb. But what good had it done? He had to admit that that smart ass Gordon had been right. He'd made no bones about the fact that interferon just didn't seem to work on lung cancer. Maybe he should have appreciated the man's honesty instead of grumbling at his uncooperativeness, which he had brought up to Lizzard.

He was 83 and was finally showing his age. The radiation, the chemotherapy and now interferon -- they hadn't done the job in the tumor, but his general appearance reflected their effects on him. What on earth would he do next?

It was time for morning rounds and unfortunately Stanley Lizzard just couldn't escape them. He didn't care much for the patient part of medicine. He was much more at ease in his office, on the phone, writing memos, or on the occasional sojourn to the laboratory to supervise his scientists and technicians as they worked on drug membrane interaction. And to make matters worse, this wasn't just any rounds. It included that Weil fellow, always pushing, pushing. Over 80, didn't he know it was time to give up and die? Can I try this? Can I try that? The man would do absolutely anything. Stanley was disgusted by his sheer desperation.

Of course the interferon hadn't worked. Now Mr. Weil wanted the newest FCI breakthrough, interleukin-2/lymphokine activated killer (IL-2/LAK) cells. Stanley had already talked to David Ryan, and it was clear that Daniel Weil was not a good candidate. And anyway, he was just one of the thousands who called in every day trying to sign up for the treatment. Ever since David's picture had appeared on the cover of Newsweek, every advanced cancer patient in the country was asking, trying to get access to IL-2. But the trial had room for only four patients per week, and each one had to be perfect. IL-2/LAK cell therapy was a very new approach in cancer treatment and everyone at the FCI was dedicated to making sure that it worked. They needed a breakthrough. Congress needed a breakthrough. The patients being treated were all very healthy-appearing with small cancers. When Weil had been told that he wasn't a good candidate, he started raising hell, calling congressmen, senators, friends all over the administration. So now they were all unhappy -- Weil, Stephen, David and Stanley all received the brunt of Weil's tirades. But they were going to stand firm on this, no matter who Mr. Weil knew. He was just too old and too sick. Patients like him could ruin their study.

The entourage entered the room. Daniel Weil looked exhausted, another night of no sleep and another day of bad news. But Stanley forged ahead.

"Well, Mr. Weil, how are you today?"

"Terrible. I didn't sleep, and I'm having pain in my chest and the damn medicine is not working. Again."

"Well, I've got some news. I talked to your doctor and we're going to transfer you back home. I'm sure you will be more comfortable there."

"And what will I do there?" Mr. Weil asked condescendingly.

"I think your oncologist should start on another regimen of chemotherapy."

"No. I don't want any more of that. All it does is make me sicker, and it doesn't work. At least when the interferon didn't work, the side effects weren't so bad." Daniel's voice still retained it's old vigor but there was the slightest suggestion of a whine, as if he knew he had come to the end of the influence line.

"I'm sorry Mr. Weil, but we've done all we can. The arrangements are final and your doctor is expecting you to be transferred home tomorrow. This is the last time I'll see you on rounds, and I want to wish you good luck." With that, Stanley reached out to shake his patient's hand, but Daniel simply turned to the wall, trying to control his mounting rage. It was okay to give him interferon, because they had nothing to lose. But this IL-2/LAK cells business was another story, because he could screw up their carefully planned experiment. Well, he wasn't going to finish with a polite handshake.

Stanley just shrugged, and led his group out of the room. As the clinical associates approached the next room, Stanley begged off, telling his assistant to continue because he needed to be in his office for an important meeting.

In truth, Stanley hadn't been feeling well himself and being in the claustrophobic hospital room seemed to intensify his uneasy sense of apprehension. As he left the hospital, that same strange sweat popped out suddenly on his forehead and under his arms. And the fevers were weird too, occurring nearly every night. There's nothing worse than a doctor with symptoms. He'd also noticed a single, swollen lymph node in his groin, and a peculiar pimple on his thigh. Could they be connected? Probably some sort of viral infection. And he'd been so damned tired and run down lately. He was only 44. No way he could be deadly sick. His pulse raced as he contemplated the possibility of having cancer. He knew he'd have to have these odd symptoms checked out soon.

Once at his building, he got into the elevator for the short ride up to the fourth floor. The familiar sense of panic enveloped him, even though the elevator was empty and the ride brief. He remembered the suffocating long elevator rides at the Cornell Medical Center in New York. And how his usual panic was intensified by these damned sweats and fevers.

He wondered what it could be.

CHAPTER 21

COCKTAILS FOR CANCER

Summer 1985

John J. Owens continued to try to run, but it wasn't easy. He could feel his enlarged liver on the right, and the jogging sometimes caused the ache to worsen. But he felt he must go on, must exercise and do as much as he could for himself. He was feeling a little better these days, now that he was over the side effects of the latest chemotherapy. He reached down to feel the funny little button under his skin through which the drugs were sent into his diseased liver. He liked to think that he now had two bellybuttons.

How could any cancer cells be left, he wondered, after all he'd been through? Surgery, systemic chemotherapy, now this direct shunt into his liver. And radiotherapy, they said, wouldn't work at all. The only thing left was research, the projects that his Task Force had funded.

John J. Owens was probably the most researched person in the United States by 1985. His Task Force had spent $3 million in 1984 funding research in colon cancer. They knew everything there was to know about the epidemiology and natural history of the disease. But now it was time to refocus. John J. had told them that morning in no uncertain terms that knowing which types of fiber to eat was wonderful, but what he wanted, what he desperately needed, was a treatment, something to squelch his cancer now, and help others in the future.

"That's a lot easier said that done," Chet Carpenter had answered. "You're funding research at four universities, two of which are leading cancer centers. We can't do much better than that. Their drugs come from the FCI, and frankly, none of them looks very promising. You can get interferon by pushing some buttons, but from what we've learned, that won't help much. And even you can't get into the FCI IL-2/LAK cell trial because you're too old and have massive disease of the liver. They only consider ex-Olympic athletes with tiny lung nodules."

"But it's my understanding that IL-2/LAK cell therapy hasn't been tested on many cancer types yet, and they're looking to expand. Isn't colon cancer an obvious direction? What about university trials? There must be trials there for colon cancer using IL-2/LAK?"

"I might be able to get you in at the University of Texas. But I must warn you that the published evidence on the treatment doesn't bode well for patients with colon cancer. I'm afraid we're about out of options. All we can do is to continue to fund basic research, and follow what's out there," Carpenter concluded.

"Hold on. What about this Salla fellow at the FCI? Didn't we hear something about him isolating a virus that causes colon cancer? I realize it isn't published yet, but couldn't we follow up on it? Do I have to go hire Dr. Salla and bring him into a research program to gain access to what he's found?" Owens asked, hardly ready to give up.

"Well, that's one way to do it, but I'm sure the price would have to be very high. Salla's budget is well over $20 million per year. He's their golden boy. Anyway, I don't see how his work will help you. It may help Roger Salla win the Nobel Prize, but it's not going to do anything in the short term for your cancer or anyone else's. It's just like the lymphoma virus announcement. Another great discovery which puts a log of money in the public coffers, but the short term practical applications for patients are nil," Carpenter said.

"Well, what then? What's next? John J. bellowed as he looked around the table. His gaze rested on a slight redhaired young man with abundant freckles. One of the younger members of the Task Force, barely out of medical school, but he brought an enthusiasm and an open mind to the proceedings that was appreciated by all. Again and again, he had questioned spending money on standard approaches, doing the same thing tomorrow that was done yesterday. He seemed more focused than the others, more concerned with finding immediate solutions to Mr. Owen's problem.

"I'd like Dr. Sheldon to give the committee a report on an inquiry he's been making. I think it will be of interest. Dr. Sheldon..." John J. announced.

The young physician stood and began setting up a slide projector, then looked about a little nervously. "I want to show a brief series of slides to illustrate a couple of technical points," he began. He flipped quickly through about 10 slides illustrating the cancer cell membrane, with close-ups of protein antigens sticking out from the cell surface. He explained that in several laboratories, mice were being immunized against antigens found on colon cancer cells, but not on most normal cells. The antibodies made by the mice could then, at least theoretically, be used to attack the colon cancer cells, with the bonus of avoiding healthy cells.

As he flicked off the projector, he summarized, "I think there are now five to ten different antibodies that react preferentially with colon cancer cells. It seems logical to me that some of these might be used in treatment."

"In mice or humans?"

"Humans, of course," replied Sheldon.

The presentation had obviously captured John J.'s attention. He looked at all the members of the Task Force for their reactions. "Well, what about it? Have they been used in treatment anywhere? What are the results? Have any of the patients responded? How long have they lived? Has anybody been cured? What do you think? Where do I sign up?"

"Hold it, hold it. What I'm trying to tell you is that these antibodies have just been made. Many researchers are busy characterizing them, trying to see which parts of their molecular make-up allow them to home in on the cancer cells. The work hasn't even been published yet, and use in treatment is only beginning. The early results are not impressive, but fewer than 60 patients have been treated using naked antibody. I suspect conjugation with a drug or other toxic substance will be required for clinical success," Sheldon said.

"Well, what are we waiting for? Let's do it. Find out who, where, how, etc. And do it now," John J. concluded with greater enthusiasm than he'd shown in quite some time.

"I'd like to suggest an alternative approach. I think it is time for you to go see Dr. Gordon," Sheldon suggested.

It was not the first time Robert Gordon's name had come before the Task Force. Earlier in John J.'s illness, he had spoken to Drs. Musso, Lizzard and Salla at the FCI, had even visited for an examination. Dr. Gordon's name had come up several times, but he just hadn't gotten around to seeing him. After all, Musson and Lizzard didn't seem to like the man very much and the two major projects he had headed up at the FCI, interferon and thymosin, hadn't really worked very well. So John J. Owens had returned to Texas, determined to find the cure by pushing the university system.

But he'd found that although the universities were more than happy to take his money and were well qualified to do research, they had trouble concentrating on his personal problem. Many times an academic laboratory group would send him glowing reports of how promising their approach was, and inevitably several months later he would be disappointed that nothing had turned up. John J. knew how the game was played. They used his money to get their laboratories up and running, and then they would apply for government grants to continue their research, veering increasingly away from work on the colon cancer cells Owens had sent along with his money. They were interested in writing papers and expanding their laboratories, not helping a sick man. He had put a stop to that.

Considering his growing frustration with the response from the academic community, Dr. Gordon's Cancer Therapeutics

Inc. was beginning to sound more attractive each day. After all, the very name echoed precisely what he was looking for. Owens wondered if they could really help him, or if this was just some scheme to make another physician wealthy. He'd have to find out.

"Dr. Sheldon, could you tell us more about Dr. Gordon's operation?"

"He has set up a controversial enterprise in Georgia which appears to be unique. He is looking at each patient's cancer as a highly individual entity, and has just begun to make combinations of antibodies -- what he calls "cocktails" -- tailored to fit a person's specific cancer, based upon those cell surface protein patterns I showed you a few minutes ago. He firmly believes that individualized treatment using the patient's own cancer as the target is the way to go."

"What do others think of the approach? What does the FCI have to say?" Owens asked, busily scribbling notes.

"Well, the concept is relatively new, and right now it's little more than Dr. Gordon's hypothesis. But I don't have to tell you about the man's reputation in the area of cancer treatment. He seems to have an unusual combination of savvy in the laboratory and at bedside. He really is an incredible man."

"Does the FCI support his ideas?"

"Not really. Dr. Lizzard is on record as saying antibodies for specific patients is a lot of baloney. Dr. Musso says high quality research can't be done in the private sector."

"I didn't like that Lizzard fellow much. I remember he looked at me kind of strangely," John J. interjected.

"On the other hand, there are firm data from Stanford indicating that anti-idiotypic antibodies are indeed patient specific for lymphoma. The question is -- are other cancers more like or more unlike one another?" Dr. Sheldon continued.

Owens seemed a little confused by the terminology, but before he could ask questions he was distracted by Chet Carpenter. "Getting back to Dr. Gordon. I've known him for years, and I can attest that he is honest, direct and pursues his own belief systems. He is one of the few people I know who hasn't been changed by the government research machine. He spent nearly a decade at the FCI, yet continues to think independently and to pursue research in an innovative manner."

"Sounds like those qualities may be why he left," John J. ventured.

"You're probably right. And now he wants to bring the research directly to patients. That is a novel approach. The government has funded and universities have conducted most cancer research to date. Add in the ACS and pharmaceutical companies and you have had an interesting little club. The Wall Street Journal has called this group the "Research Regulatory Alliance" with the FDA participating as the approval point for new drugs. With the ante $100 million to participate in the development of each drug, they have a nice little monopoly. I think you should go see him. Hell John J., if you're going to fund research, this place looks like it was created just for you! Research for the individual. Give it a shot!" Carpenter said passionately.

John J. Owens practically danced on the table. "Absolutely. Chet, since you know him, why don't you set up an appointment with Dr. Gordon as soon as possible, and I want the cell lines and frozen tumor cells transferred to his laboratory immediately. Let's see what he can do." And he practically bolted from the room in his excitement.

As John J. stopped to get a drink, he absentmindedly stroked the little artificial belly button. *Maybe they can stick an antibody cocktail in here and fix me up!*

CHAPTER 22

SUSPICION

Spring 1985

"Ladies and gentlemen, I'm pleased to announce the awarding of the 1985 Wilson Prize to Dr. Stephen Musso, director of the prestigious Federal Cancer Institute."

As Stephen stood and walked to the podium, applause broke out in ripples, building to a crescendo and a standing ovation. The Wilson Prize was the most coveted science award in the United States, and he was the only man ever to have received it twice. First for his ABC combination chemotherapy, and now for the discovery of the lymphoma virus. Well, ABC hasn't led to the Nobel, but maybe this one will, he thought as he climbed the marble steps to the platform.

Stephen gazed out over the audience, some 500 strong -- Influential people from across America. Many of his family were standing in the front rows. He spotted several enemies at the periphery and in the back, men whose careers he had endeavored to "restructure" for various reasons. But the vast majority were neither friend nor enemy, just working scientists and their spouses who recognized him for the leader he was, the most powerful single figure in American science. He not only dispensed $1.5 billion of public money yearly, but he and his colleagues (some said henchmen) determined the direction of every major effort in cancer research. Personally, he was a man who favored his few friends and punished his growing list of enemies. And so the applause coming from the audience was not from joy or friendship or even respect, but of fear and in not a few cases, frustration or anger.

"Ladies and gentlemen, I want to thank the Wilson committee and all of you for your support in the award of this honor. I must say, though, a great deal of credit goes to my colleagues. I am but a simple clinician, a man interested primarily in patient treatment. You have seen fit to help me help others through the directorship of the Federal Cancer Institute, but there is little I could have done without your support and assistance, and there is little I could have done in the discovery of this important virus without the help of my colleagues in the laboratory."

Roger Salla, seated at the center table from which Stephen had just arisen, nearly choked on the cracker he was grinding between his back teeth to keep from screaming, or perhaps crying. The lymphoma virus was his discovery, and he was not the only one in the room who knew it. Stephen could blather on ad nauseum about his wonderful colleagues, would even name names, and he sure as hell wouldn't split any of the prize money or convey any of the recognition.

But Roger would have his day. Musso may have won the Wilson Prize twice, Roger smirked, but the announcement of his colon cancer virus would knock the socks off the scientific community. That's the one that people will remember. And it's all mine, and I'll do anything and everything to see that it stays that way.

Stephen droned on, recounting for the zillionth time his accomplishments in the chemotherapy of lymphoma. He dramatically and movingly described the sequence of events leading to the discovery of the ABC regimen, went on to summarize the pathophysiology of lymphoma, often using first names to cleverly create a sense of "being there" and ending with an almost passionate recounting of the discovery of HLV-1. It was quite an exciting tale of scientific detective work.

Unfortunately, very little of it was true.

It didn't fit at all with the facts as remembered by Adrian Free and Tom Frederick, by Paulo Brazella, George Trumpey or Roger Salla. But it was the public version, the one that

Stephen told and perfected at the 80 or more events each year where he was asked to speak, spreading the word of his greatness at major gatherings of scientists as well as to prestigious lay groups. And like an error in a standard textbook that is perpetuated in later volumes, to the point that everyone accepts it as fact, Stephen Musso's conquest of lymphoma was believed by many to be absolute fact. Didn't the Wilson Prize -- two Wilson Prizes -- prove it?

Later that evening, alone in his study, Stephen was worried. On the surface all appeared to be going well. This year's grant strategy was working, the FCI contract system continuing to support the "right" people. His system of disbursement of public monies to support his friends and valued colleagues was running as smoothly as ever. The chemotherapy development program continued to prosper, and there was an unending line of new drugs in the pipeline. By restructuring the biotherapy program he now had it functioning smoothly under Lou Brody in the clinical center in Washington and he'd gotten rid of that troublesome do-gooder Robert Gordon. All was indeed well within the FCI and its university community.

But his sensors were up. There was just a hint of a problem.

Sam Fish had recently fired a post-doctoral scientist named Martin Bartholomew, who had worked in the laboratory of viral oncology. He'd been there for two years and would probably have begun looking for an industrial or academic position within the year, and then he'd be gone, a normal turn of events for a post-doc. Normally, Stephen wouldn't bother himself about the fate of such an underling, but this Bartholomew fellow had worried him.

He was a snoop.

He was asking questions about George Trumpey's site visit. He was very curious about the amount of internal support and outside contract funding for Roger Salla's work. And he took more than the average virologist's interest in the HLV-1 story and in Roger's possible virus for colon cancer. He simply asked far too many questions and the last episode had been particularly disturbing.

Sam had grown suspicious of Bartholomew's frequent questions, so he had one of his staff go through the post- doc's desk and office files late one night. And the search had been most revealing. One of Bartholomew's drawers was stuffed full of photocopies of FCI contracts, memoranda, letters, notes and agendas. It was a great deal of material that was clearly outside the bounds of a post-doc.

Sam had fired him the next day, assuring Stephen that as a junior scientist, there was no way that Bartholomew could possibly have access to anything really damaging. But Stephen wasn't so sure, and was having second thoughts about Sam's action. Bartholomew didn't need classified documents to piece together the basics of Stephen's philosophy. And there were certainly ex-FCI people out there who could corroborate Bartholomew's suspicions. How did they know that the snoop didn't have copies of everything in his apartment?

Stephen had been fearful of just such a problem ever since the Washington Post investigation of FCI management several years ago. Those two reporters had come dangerously close to understanding his real management system. Fortunately for him, the reporters had chosen to focus on drug toxicity in children, thereby incurring the wrath of pediatric oncologists and families who believed they were attacking a system dedicated to fighting disease in children. Stephen knew their investigation would have been far more damaging had they pursued his reward and punishment system.

And there was that peculiar episode with Connie. They had repeatedly been together for the last four years. Always in his apartment or hers, never out in public. She was warm and supportive and at the same time was an animal in bed. He didn't "love" her, not as he did his wife and family, but he needed her, lusted after her, used her and she never questioned him. Until four weeks ago. He had found her crying in her apartment, very upset, not willing to talk about whatever it was that disturbed her. But he had been surprised when she told him that, after nearly a decade in the government, she was leaving. Taking a public relations position with a mid-sized pharmaceutical company in Florida. It was a good opportunity, more pay, more prestige; a real coup for Connie. Then why the tears? He had assumed it was about leaving him. Women! Hard to understand.

She couldn't know about Melody, and he had never revealed any "hidden truths" about himself to her. She did have full access to his apartment. No real reason to worry. just strange that these problems with Bartholomew and Connie had occurred at the same time. It was probably nothing, Stephen told himself. And Connie had written a brief note. She was settled and happy in Florida. No invitation to come visit. But still, he was uneasy -- a feeling of unrest that even two Wilson prizes couldn't stem.

CHAPTER 23

PRIVATE RESEARCH

Fall 1985

If ever there was a scientific term that ought to be renamed, this was it. "Anti-idiotypic antibody." Senator Tomasi couldn't even pronounce it, let along begin to understand it. Yet it just might be what would save his life.

It was funny how everyone still called him Senator. He had not run for re-election and had not served in public office for three years. Yet, he was still the ever-popular Senator Tomasi. He was at home now in Connecticut, and feeling quite well. His lymphoma had responded to treatment, and his lymph nodes were almost imperceptible.

But he knew this suspended sentence wouldn't last long. And so he had done everything reasonable to prepare for the eventuality of the cancer's return. He looked back over the past three years with some satisfaction, for he'd covered every available base. He had visited the best facility in the East, the Dana-Farber Center in Boston. He'd consulted with the top physicians at the prestigious Sloan-Kettering, M.D. Anderson, and UCLA medical centers. By now he could get up and lecture about surgery, radiotherapy, and multiple forms of chemotherapy with an astounding amount of specific knowledge on his cancer. Tomasi's wealth had enabled him to go one step farther than most patients though, in the form of a full-time physician on his staff, who kept him abreast on virtually all new developments in cancer research. His doctor had investigated bone marrow transplants, interferon, interleukin-2, monoclonal antibodies, and now these anti-idiotypic antibodies.

Robert Tomasi was all set to meet the future, with pieces of himself stashed away in important laboratories here and there. He had his bone marrow in storage at Dana-Farber in case high dose "chemo" and a bone marrow transplant was needed some day. He was looking into a human cell bank in New Jersey, to see if they would literally put his diseased tissue on ice for whatever treatments might arise in the years to come. Chunks of his lymph nodes had been sent to Dr. Hertzog at Stanford and Dr. Gordon at the FCI so that research on his tissue could continue even though the chemotherapy appeared to have been effective, at least for the present. Both investigators had promised to try to make anti-idiotypic antibodies for him, but progress was slow, and recent reports were disturbing.

Last week, Dr. Hertzog had called with "final" results, which turned out to be no results at all. He simply had not been able to make the antibody, something about his cancer cells not making enough of their own peculiar idiotype to do the immunizations. The Senator didn't fully understand the process, even with his physician's explanations, but he grasped that somehow his lymphoma cells should produce an unusual sort of antibody, and if that antibody could be captured and his cells coaxed to grow in the laboratory, then these anti-idiotype antibodies could be made against it. These anti-antibodies would then somehow be able to destroy the tumor cells that carried his original odd antibodies on their surfaces. He understood that antibody molecules looked a little like upright lobsters protruding out from his cancer cells, with different types having different patterns of indentations on the claws. The anti-idiotype antibodies would "fit" the claw pattern of the antibodies that dotted his tumor cells, and could be used as a homing device of sorts, particularly if they could be hooked up to a cancer-fighting drug. This was all terrific, except that Dr. Hertzog couldn't even get a handle on the first step, harnessing the little rascals dangling from his cancer cells.

But how hard was he trying? Tomasi's staff had advised him that Dr. Hertzog was unquestionably a leader in university research on this therapy, but this very fact could be hindering his progress. The man was simply too busy to be much concerned with the cells of one man, even if that man was a public figure. And the goal of his laboratory, of any academic laboratory, was research and publications; a larger laboratory; more money; recognition. If some poor soul happened to benefit directly from that research, well, that was wonderful. But it wasn't the overriding goal.

Senator Tomasi wanted to be that goal. He wanted research to cure his personal problem. First the cure, with public recognition, then back to politics and his quest for the Presidency.

But he also had his proverbial foot in another door, that of the FCI. Isn't that what his consulting physicians always said? Go to the FCI. And he had. But he didn't fit the requirements for any ongoing trials, and he wasn't the sort of person to throw his influence around if it meant some other cancer patient would be bumped from his spot. Anyway, none of those trials had the goal of cure he desired. At least his influence had persuaded the hot shots to speak with him, and they had introduced him to Dr. Robert Gordon. He came very highly praised, a man of great foresight and compassion who was leading the FCI biotherapy program to a truly world class effort. And Dr. Gordon had been most pleasant, suggesting that the senator send a sample of his lymph node tissue to his laboratory. Because Gordon's was the only serious program doing this type of research besides Hertzog's, Tomasi had arranged to have the tissue sent immediately. Between Hertzog and Gordon, he thought, something would certainly come out of it.

But he hadn't counted on politics. FCI politics, that is.

The highly-respected Dr. Gordon had quite suddenly departed the Institute, under rather vague circumstances, something to do with policy. And what had become of Senator Tomasi's lymph node sample in all this? No one seemed to know. One thing was sure, the (his) antibody project was no longer "top priority."

Being a Senator had given him some understanding of the politics of government and politics of science. He guessed that Robert Gordon had been a little too independent and vocal, and hadn't played the subservient role on the team led by Stephen Musso. But whatever Gordon's personal beef with the government honchos, his dismissal presented a gap in Tomasi's research project. So he had personally gone to Georgia to speak with Dr. Gordon. As far as Robert knew, the federal antibody project was to continue but he had no information on recent progress; and, he had no control over current and future events in his old program.

But Tomasi had been able to get further information from some old friends, and like the Hertzog story, the answer was that there was no progress. His tissue had been frozen away for posterity, and was not being examined or used for anything. The FCI laboratories had gotten involved in the AIDS and Kaposi's sarcoma work, pushing his run-of-the-mill lymphoma aside. And after all, he was no longer a Senator.

Now Robert Gordon was championing private sector support of cancer research. So he had been on the mark when he had suspected Gordon's renegade tendencies, Tomasi thought. Although the corporate approach to privatization of research had disquieting features for a liberal Democratic ex-Senator from Connecticut, a man who had dedicated himself to finding a better system of support for the 35 million uninsured patients in the United States, it did have some intriguing features. And, in his current situation, the value of the novel approach was obvious.

If you put aside the restrictive nature and the cost of a pay-for-service enterprise, Tomasi thought, the total dedication to a particular individual was certainly something unique. Bringing the research laboratory directly to bear on the individual patient also made sense. Plus, he liked Dr. Gordon personally, especially the fact that he wanted each of his patients to actively participate in the project by being as informed as possible. Tomasi's experience on the Science and

Technology Senate subcommittee had come in handy in this regard. He'd even be able to explain anti-idiotype antibodies soon.

Perhaps most convincing of all was the huge effort being put forth on behalf of biotherapy. No longer an unpopular quirky theory, treating cancer with the body's own chemicals was not big business. Wall Street investment banking firms were not scrambling to hire not just top-notch MBAs, but MBAs with Ph.D.s in molecular biology. More than 200 biotechnology companies had mushroomed onto the scene, with as many as 100 of them working on approaches for the treatment of cancer. Major pharmaceutical and chemical companies were spinning off or buying biotech departments and subsidiaries right and left. Considering the headliners such as interferon, interleukin-2 and antibodies, plus the still rather mysterious colony stimulating factors and tumor necrosis factor, hundreds of new approaches in cancer biotherapy were likely to be available in the next decade, if not sooner.

What on earth would the FDA do, Tomasi wondered. Now, at best, the system had only three or four drugs wending their way through the FDA maze yearly, with usually a lone new drug approval each year, if that. Wasn't it obvious that this system couldn't handle the influx of new biological substances for cancer treatment? The FDA was actually shrinking in size without any increase in efficiency during a time when the input number of new medicines from biotechnology companies was dramatically increasing. It was a system in which change was needed. Maybe Gordon's company, Cancer Therapeutics, could help lighten the load, or at least speed things up. Robert Gordon's view that the FDA approval process would have to evolve to keep up with the new biology, rather than try to squeeze a bigger foot into an old shoe, made perfect sense. And so did the private-focused approach on an individual human being.

For ex-Senator and lymphoma patient Robert Tomasi, Cancer Therapeutics was clearly the way to go. He would have yet another lymph node biopsy sent to Georgia.

He had a feeling that this time the lymph node would not be lost in the shuffle.

CHAPTER 24

ROUNDS

Spring 1986

Good Samaritan Hospital was abuzz with excitement. Everything seemed to be happening at once in the facility tucked away in the beautiful, rolling hills of Fairfield, on the north side of Atlanta. It all centered around the large laboratory building going up for Cancer Therapeutics, under construction adjacent to the hospital. The outpatient clinic on the first two floors was nearly complete. Soon CTI would leave its primitive temporary quarters and move to a modern laboratory and clinic equal to any university or government institution.

Funding for CTI had been successful, and the concept of privatization and the new role of the research laboratory as a clinical resource was attracting intense media scrutiny. Dr. Gordon had displayed an uncanny talent at being interviewed and convincing people of the merits of his groundbreaking approach to cancer treatment. So far he had been on the "Today Show," the "CBS Evening News" and "60 Minutes." Write-ups had appeared in Time, Newsweek, the New York Times and the Wall Street Journal. The controversial CTI was focusing much attention on Good Samaritan.

A 400 bed general medical and surgical hospital, Good Samaritan had enjoyed a good reputation in the mid South region for many years. But never before had Good Sam undertaken a research effort; it had simply excelled in delivering standard medical/surgical care. But in the tumult of the late 1970s, the Sisters had made what was to be an excellent long term decision. They had put into place a professional management team to run the hospital, taking themselves out of day-to-day management and operations. And they convinced their board to leave Central Atlanta to build a new hospital in suburban Fairfield.

The decision had been a sound one. Things went so well that by 1982, a gleaming new hospital was dedicated, a facility built for the year 2000. The outpatient clinic was of a size usually seen with a 1,000 bed hospital. The inpatient component was smaller and more efficient, considering the onrushing DRG system. And the northward growth of Atlanta placed the hospital in the center of the largest population center of professionals, corporate executives, lawyers and physicians in the United States.

The Sisters had also made the rather radical decision to support and nurture Dr. Gordon's program of privatization. Considerable controversy surrounded the initiation of this program. Wasn't it research for the rich, an access system for the wealthy, to the exclusion of not only the poor, but probably the middle class as well? How could that fit with the mission of the Sisters and Good Samaritan Hospital? It was a matter of vigorous debate in 1984.

Robert Gordon had presented his case well. If we treat those patients who are rejected by public programs, he argued, how can we be judged exclusionary? The "system" had already rejected them. If we deliver research services to patients who otherwise wouldn't get them, how can that be called restricted access? If we give access to a segment of the population, isn't that better than no access at all? Isn't access to research different than access to treatment? If research becomes effective treatment, shouldn't insurance and government make it available to all?

Dr. Gordon even had an answer for the inevitable question of what to do with those who might benefit from biotherapy but who couldn't afford to fund a personal research program. Some of the media tried to paint Dr. Gordon as a bit of greedy ogre, this very question had kept him awake through many a night. And he thought he had an answer, although it wouldn't be immediate. Perhaps industry, philanthropists, and the hospitals themselves could contribute funds to assist patients who were medically qualified for research programs but financially unable to proceed.

The Sisters of Good Samaritan had been convinced, realized that the eventual acceptance of a novel research mission could ultimately enhance the hospital's reputation, which would lead to positive fallout across many programs. They were bottom-line oriented, and fully realized that revenues must exceed expenses. Beds must be filled, and if Dr. Gordon's program did that, who were they to object?

But they really hadn't expected all of this attention! Doctors from all over the country were coming to see how this research privatization worked. The same old questions were repeatedly being asked, but in a more positive framework. How did Good Sam deal with the thorny issues involved? What were their policies? Did insurance reimburse for these services? How can I do this in my hospital? Little by little, the medical community as well as the public was beginning to understand that the line-up-and-wait attitude of the government was simply not an efficient way to deal with new cancer treatments. And it certainly was not in the individual's best interest. Few could qualify as the "perfect" patient and enter a government/university clinical trial.

And finally, a few genuinely curious reporters had emerged from the rubble of those eager to throw stones. These few were addressing the questions of the cost of research. Critics focused on the high cost of CTIs programs -- but had they any idea of what similar experiments cost the taxpayer at the FCI? What the cost to patients and insurers in a university hospital? In fact, costs were actually lower in the private sector! Why couldn't private research initiatives join forces with government, university and industry programs to battle their common enemy? Diversity could only have a positive effect.

In spite of all the press hoopla and inquisitive visiting physicians, life in a hospital goes on. There are still patients, still nurses, and still needs. On this sunny May 24, 1986, Dr. Gordon was making his rounds. No longer did he lead an entourage of fellows, residents, interns, students and nurses, as he had a few miles south at Mallory. No longer the "Professor" in the finest European tradition. Those rounds were more a teaching mechanism than a patient care exercise. The pace had been so hectic that often they were neither. But here at Good Samaritan, there were only doctors, nurses and patients, and now Dr. Gordon was wending his way through his portion of the 40 beds allocated to CTI, with the head oncology nurse on ward 4B.

CTI had already grown to include five medical oncologists. Although they participated in weekly conferences, wrote papers together and discussed their problems and accomplishments on a day-to-day basis, each took care of his patients individually. And the patients came from all over the world. If their laboratory research project was successful, they went to ward 4B for treatment. So unlike most oncology wards, 4B had an aura of joy. For simply to be there meant that there was hope.

Robert always enjoyed rounds. He had 10 patients on ward 4B now, and each was a fascinating individual with a specific problem. And each needed to be approached in his or her own special way.

First on rounds was Dr. Daniel Weil, a truly amazing man. He was 85 years old and still fighting. He was a scion of the chemical industry, a man with considerable scientific expertise and of great personal wealth. He had been through the system. Surgery for lung cancer with a recurrence, postoperative radiotherapy that didn't work, combination chemotherapy with a reduction in the mass in his left lung, but with subsequent recurrence, interferon with no effect, and the final common denominator of all residents of 4B: Daniel Weil was judged too old and too sick for further experimental trials at the Federal Cancer Institute.

So he had come to Good Sam and to Dr. Gordon and had made his case well.

"Look, I'm 85 years old, and this damn tumor is pushing on the structures in the center of my chest. I've exhausted all forms of standard therapy and all the experimental treatment that I can get through the FCI/university system, but I'm not ready to quit. I want to take whatever opportunity might exist and try it. Money is no object. If you need funding for research, just tell me how much and I'll make it happen." He had been blunt and direct.

"Dr. Weil, thank you, the money will be helpful. But we will only accept it, and you of course, if you are medically able to undergo the treatment. Let's do an exam, and then we'll see where you stand," he had replied.

Daniel Weil was indeed a very sick man but not too sick to attempt one of CTIs programs. "I think perhaps we should try our Interleukin-2/activated cell program. Yes, I know you were rejected for a similar government program, but our protocol is somewhat gentler. No one your age has ever been treated with this approach, but I think you can tolerate it. How about it?"

"Let's go for it doctor. I'm ready for anything!" Daniel responded with as much enthusiasm as he could muster.

"And now for the bad news."

"Side effect, you mean? Didn't you just say your method was gentler?" Daniel said.

"Yes, we spread our IL-2 dose over time, but there are still problems, and I want you to understand them up front, it's part of the informed consent under which we conduct our studies. Most of the patients with lung cancer have, in fact, not responded to IL-2/activated cells, and most have had rather substantial side effects."

"Such as?" Daniel interjected a bit hesitantly.

"Fever, chills, fluid retention. The FCI has had more severe problems along these lines but it's not generally publicized. Many of their patients have actually gotten quite ill."

"But if the treatment stops, do they feel better?"

"Yes. But it's not terribly pleasant during the few weeks of the treatment."

"Look, I'm a veteran of anything you could possible do to a cancer patient. I can take it."

"Dr. Weil, I think you can too, or I wouldn't have suggested it. And the reason I do want you to try it is that several of our patients with adenocarcinoma of the lung indeed had substantial responses. These are still in remission some six months later. Why not give it a try?"

And Dr. Gordon's instincts had been correct. Dr. Weil had finished his round of treatment, and although there had been the anticipated side effects, he too had shown a response. His tumor had shrunk to less than half of its original volume, and his breathing had improved dramatically. Finally, he was ready for discharge.

"Dr. Weil, how are you feeling today? Ready to tackle the world again?"

"Better, much, much better, doctor. My breathing is the best it's been in six months and the pain is almost gone," the beaming patient replied.

"Well, you've had an excellent response to treatment. You're a very special man, Dr. Weil, the oldest patient ever treated with this type of biotherapy and one out of only a small number of lung cancer patients who have responded to IL-2/activated cells. And the shrinkage has been considerable."

"If there are going to be responders, I'm happy to be among them. I don't know how to thank you," Dr. Weil said.

"Don't thank me yet. Remember, this is experimental, and we can't say how long the response will last, or if it will have any long term influence on your life. But it is gratifying to see the shrinkage, and I want you to keep in contact with me so that we can monitor it."

"Will I be on chemotherapy or anything in the meantime?"

"No, I don't want to interfere with observing the results of the experimental therapy. We won't initiate further treatment unless we see regrowth of the tumor."

"That's wonderful, just wonderful. Do you know how awful it is to leave the hospital after painful treatment only to be told you must come back twice a week for more discomfort?" It's been a tough month, but I'm really looking forward to just relaxing at home with my family. I am so grateful for your allowing me to participate in this experiment. You may have just given me my life back. Keep up the great work!"

"Thank you, Dr. Weil. And you have been a good patient. Please keep in touch."

"By the way Doctor, please call me Daniel. I retired my Ph.D. degree years ago. I'll call you in a few weeks for a progress report."

Robert and Nurse Smithson put some final notes in Daniel Weil's chart and set him up for discharge. Releasing a patient from an experimental oncology ward in reasonable health was cause for celebration, for so few responded. Even if the patient's return to health was for a limited time, it could still be counted as a step in the right direction.

Lydia Green was also feeling better on this day. Her latest bout with chemotherapy seemed to be working. By the time Dr. Gordon got to her room, she had already been up and down the corridor several times.

"Good morning doctor. The chemotherapy is working! I'm feeling much better. It looks like you've given me another reprieve," she said eagerly.

"Yes Lydia, you are doing better. Your lymph nodes are shrinking and I'm pleased to tell you that the fluid in your left chest is nearly gone. It looks as though you are going back into remission."

"How long do you think it'll last this time?" she asked quietly.

"It's hard to say. Just as with the previous chemotherapy, chances are the effects will be temporary. For some patients it lasts for years, but more likely, in a few months there will be a diminishing of your response. Then most patients go on to something new."

"But what about me? Haven't I tried every something new already? It looks to me like you need to pull another rabbit out of your hat from that laboratory. I think I'm about finished with the drugs," she said.

Once again, a patient knew exactly where she stood. "Yes, you are about finished with the drugs. We've used nearly every form of chemotherapy that might work, and your bone marrow tolerance is poor. If this regimen fails, that's it, I'm afraid, for the drugs."

They both paused for a moment, each thinking the same thing. The research project. Lydia was about to ask about it when Dr. Gordon began to explain it, not wanting her to despair that all hope was lost when this final drug regimen ceased it activity.

"But there's good news from the laboratory. We have succeeded in isolating the antibody being made by your lymphoma cells, and excellent progress has been made on that anti-idiotypic antibody we discussed. I think by the time you need it, we'll have it," he said. Lydia just loved it when he smiled and now he was absolutely grinning.

Lydia watched him as he expertly evaluated her condition. The lymph nodes were noticeably smaller, the liver had shrunk, and the spleen couldn't be felt. Her bothersome skin rash was gone and the itching had diminished. Her peak temperature last week had been 100.8 degrees and night sweats were nearly gone. Yes, she was going into remission.

"Well, what can I expect from the idiot antibody?" Lydia asked as he wrote a brief note on her chart. "Will this finally be the cure?"

"Lydia, you know that I can't make that sort of projection, much as I'd like to. As I've said before, it's an insurance policy, an option for the future, a chance to try an experiment that gives you an opportunity. At worst, it will fail completely, and we'll have to try another approach. At best, yes, it might arrest the cancer. For now though, let's hope this remission lasts for several months or even years, and when and if your tumor returns, we'll try the antibody and hope for the best."

"I know, I know. Just another guinea pig. Well, I'm pretty used to it by now. But this time, at least, the treatment is specific for this guinea pig, and I know you'll do your best." She reached out and gave him a hug.

Robert enjoyed seeing Mr. Owens on rounds. He was such a dynamic man, such a ball of fire. How could a cancer dare to grow in his body, Robert often wondered. He asked such incredibly intuitive questions. He and Sam Luria together probably knew more about cancer than most physicians. Certainly, they knew a great deal about their individual problems and the potential solutions. They read and studied almost nonstop, and the nurses assigned to them had to be strong to carry the medical journals back and forth to the library downstairs. They ought to just open a branch in their rooms.

Both men were also addicted to the telephone. Robert often thought of putting them in the same room with only one phone and seeing what happened. Sam Luria would probably win for the phone was literally his lifeline. He didn't have the financial resources that Owens did, whose private task force did much of the phoning.

"How are you doing this morning, John J.?" Robert asked as he entered the sunny room. He addressed most patients formally, but the robust Texan had insisted on informality from the beginning. Like Lydia Green, Robert felt a special closeness to the man, and the familiarity just seemed right.

"Much better. I can feel those mice you gave me running around inside my body. They're eating up those tumor cells right and left."

Robert laughed. "Well, that's an interesting way to describe your treatment. You're right though, the antibodies are indeed from mice, and I hope they are running around ferreting out your tumor cells. There is no question that something is happening. With just six injections of the antibody hooked to the chemotherapy drug, Mitomycin C, your liver is already shrinking. This is particularly exciting because chemotherapy is not generally very useful against colon cancer. It looks as if it may work differently when hooked to antibody." Robert had a tendency to forget that he was talking to a patient, so knowledgeable was John J., and he often went into rambling explanations of the cancer's response.

"Well, I hope you're right Doc. I know my liver doesn't hurt like hell it used to. You keep right on giving me those treatments right through my button," he said as he pointed rather proudly to the catheter entry site near his umbilicus, his second bellybutton.

"Your CT scan was downright exhilirating -- your liver is half the size it was when it was when you entered Good Samaritan. John J., I have high hopes for your antibody cocktail. Now, what about side effects? Feel anything?"

"You mean besides my urge to chow down a huge side of barbeque? No. I feel better every day. Nothing like the side effects of chemotherapy. How about that Doc?"

"Well, Mitomycin C is a much more toxic drug than the 5-FU and FUdR you've failed. It seems likely that the antibody is targeting the drug to your tumor cells and protecting the healthy cells from toxicity. That's the way we intended it to work, and it's gratifying to see that happen."

"Doc, I'm thrilled to see the experiment going my way. When can I go home?"

"In about two weeks. I want to finish this series of injections using the mouse antibodies. We may not be able to give them to you again, so I want to inject the maximum dose during this first series," Dr. Gordon responded.

"What? What will I do if they stop working? I thought that only was supposed to happen with conventional chemotherapy."

"As you know, John J., this is all experimental. For now we are using mice to manufacture the antibodies, and some patients develop allergic reactions because the antibody does not come from humans. But while you are still tolerating the mouse antibody, we are working on developing human monoclonal antibodies for you. This is where your research project funding is primarily going."

"Wow, this is like being part of Star Wars or something. I just hope it works."

"So do I, John J. So do I." Robert said as he rose and patted his patient on the shoulder.

As Robert left the room, he felt a great deal of satisfaction with his patient and the shrinking tumor. Here was a man who had lived life right, had kept himself in good shape, had prospered in business, made many contributions to society, then bang, he had been struck by disaster in the prime of life. He had done everything he could to deal with it, but had found the government and universities wanting. And now here he was participating in the CTI approach. Robert hoped John J.'s progress would continue.

Next, Robert weaved in and out of several rooms, seeing patients in for a variety of treatments -- monoclonal antibody immunoconjugates, Interleukin-2/activated cells, infusions of activated macrophages into the abdominal cavity, specific immunotherapy with vaccines made from their tumor cells, and other biological approaches. Finally, he was doing things the way it felt best, patient by patient, disease by disease, using the laboratory to practice medicine.

The last room on the right belonged to Sam Luria, the chatterbox. Sam was in the hospital for restaging. He really wasn't having much difficulty, wasn't even currently under treatment. His blood protein level had been stable for two years now, and except for his mild bone pain, he had really done quite well. There was some scoliosis in his back from the collapse of certain vertebrae, which made it difficult for him to get around. Otherwise, he was in fairly good shape. Occasional punched out holes in the bones were seen in X-ray, and his bone scan was still positive. But the myeloma appeared to be reasonably quiescent over the last three years since the Alkeran and Prednisone had been discontinued. Mr. Luria was in the hospital now for a bone marrow and re-evaluation and things looked pretty good.

"Good morning Mr. Luria, how are you doing today?" Robert asked.

"Great, I feel just great! I did my usual five flights of stairs, and burned up the hallways yesterday, and I'm gonna do the same today. I've also been on the telephone."

"Really?" Robert said with a chuckle. Mr. Luria was AT&T's best friend.

"Have you heard about beta glucouronidase? I understand that enzyme is elevated in patients with multiple myeloma. Do you think it has anything to do with immunoglobulin expression on the cell membrane?"

That question would have sounded unusual had it come from any patient other than Mr. Luria or perhaps John J. Owens, but Robert had learned that this little guy was an amazing storehouse of information. His daily telephone bill rivaled his hospital bill. Sam Luria was a restauranteur of moderate means, not a rich man like John J. or Daniel Weil, but he was more aggressive than both of them put together. He used the telephone as his own modality of cancer treatment, calling doctor after doctor, laboratory after laboratory, and hospitals one after another. By doing this, he systematically extracted information from multiple sources and synthesized it in his mind. The man seemed to have a photographic memory and nothing was actually written down except for a few scraggly notes he kept by his telephone. True, he sometimes got his facts mixed up, and he often put an inappropriate value on a source of information. Overall, however, the result was that he knew more about multiple myeloma than most physicians. He even knew more about it than some oncologists. So every day on rounds, when he came to Sam Luria, Robert was prepared for an extended question and answer period. It was a new form of "teaching rounds!"

For this question, like many, he had to think a moment. "Well, I don't know, Mr. Luria. There are indeed changes in that particular enzyme, but it's not clear what it has to do with antibody secretion. As you know, it's difficult to measure because the assay is not very reliable."

Sam thought for a moment. "Okay, but what about my antibodies doctor? Are you making any progress there?"

"Let's keep pushing, Mr. Luria. You know the system only responds when you push."

"What do you mean? What is the problem?" he asked.

"The problem is a bit ironic. You're doing too well."

"Huh? I know you've explained this before, but it is confusing."

"Well, your bone marrow has a sparse population of myeloma cells, enough to give that positive bone scan. But there are also many healthy cells, which is why you feel a little better. We may not be able to extract enough myeloma cells to provoke an antibody response in the mouse. Plus, the healthy cells might also immunize the mouse. We'd end up with a whole bunch of different antibodies, not all of which would react where we want them to. So we have to go to existing hybridomas, from other patients, while we continue to try to make one from your cells."

"So how is the search going?"

"I've been checking on your project every day. So far we've been able to locate five hybridomas making different antibodies from three different universities. Now we have to see if they react with your myeloma cells, which is why we took the bone marrow today. If we can produce those hybridomas, your project will really speed up."

"I know, but it's so frustrating! These antibodies you're checking were made with FCI funding, using taxpayer dollars, made at three different universities, by three different investigators. I've spoken to them all, but still we can't get the hybridomas. What's going on? What good is government funded research if you can't use the results? I'm calling my congressman and senator today. Maybe some political action will make things happen," Sam said defiantly as he eyed the phone.

"I agree. I think you ought to proceed along those lines. You're absolutely right. The antibodies should be available. Those institutions have been discussing their release for six months now, and they continue to discuss it. But I think I know the real problem, which you may not have suspected."

"Yes?" Mr. Luria prompted.

"It's economics. They think the hybridomas have commercial value, and they are afraid that if they're shipped out, they'll lose control over the economics. However, having made them with public money, they should be available to you as a taxpayer and as a patient. Let's both keep pushing."

"Economics? When my life is at stake? It's all very hard to believe. I thought they were criticizing you on economics? But yes, I'll keep pushing, maybe drum up some political action. Plus, the patient committees I've set up are growing all over the United States. Even if they can't help me, the movement to organize patients to deal with these logistical problems will certainly help those in the future. Patients must become more active in their own care. The problem is that cancer patients die too soon to work on their own problem. Hey, I have an idea! Keep me alive so I can make this patient organization work!" Sam smiled.

"Mr. Luria, if a telephone can make it happen, you're the best man for the job," Robert smiled broadly and left the room.

CHAPTER 25

WARHEADS AND COCKTAILS

Summer 1986

Robert Gordon called in his whole team to go over some recent results from the laboratory. Decisions had to be made.

"I don't have to tell you how important this particular project is," he began, barely able to conceal his excitement. "All of you know the patients for whom we do research. Many of them have toured our laboratory to let you know that it is them in the petrie dish, so I know you're all conscious of the importance of each project and each patient. However, we can't ignore the fact that this particular patient could have a broader impact on our work than any other. Many of our patients are wealthy and influential, but Senator Tomasi is the one with the most public recognition. Although our research for him is only known within his family and within our team, if we're successful, it will surely attract a great deal of positive attention to our enterprise. Now, I say this not to have you approach his lymph node any differently than you would anyone else's, but I just want you to be aware of the potential impact of his research and the treatment program."

Everyone nodded. Anyway you cut it, they were a public entity with stockholders and a unique position in the public eye with respect to their patients. It was mid 1986 and they had been in operation for more than a year. And it was becoming clear that they were indeed making progress. Their first paper had been published in the prestigious New England Journal of Medicine.

The scientific community was beginning to recognize that CTI, a small privately financed venture that had just gone public, was more than the hare-brained idea of Robert Gordon, disgruntled FCI investigator. The focus on Dr. Gordon, Good Samaritan Hospital, and CTI continued, and as predicted by Bill Toban, the recent public stock offering had been a huge success, raising new capital in excess of $50 million for the company. There was no longer any question of the concept. Now it was a matter of depth and scope. Could it work for a few? Might it work for many? For all cancer patients?

CTI was having real success in its aggressive research program on understanding and treating lymphoma. And Senator Tomasi's tumor was proving amenable to a daring new treatment approach. Dick Belner went to the blackboard and outlined a series of experiments done for the Senator.

"We've isolated his tumor cell antibody, the immunoglobulin made by his lymphoma cells. As all of you know, Dr. Hertzog at Stanford attempted this over two years ago, and failed. Now, it may be that we are better at isolating these antibodies, or it may be that the new biopsy provided better material. I suspect the former," he chuckled, "but I'm sure Dr. Hertzog would focus the latter."

"Anyway, we've proceeded to immunize a series of mice, and we now have five antibodies which react with these lymphoma cells. I am quite pleased to announce that the cocktail is ready to be administered. Now, the unique thing about this particular treatment is that we have loaded the antibodies with different drugs. All the previous patients have been treated with a single drug such as Adriamycin or Mitomycin C loaded on the antibody cocktail. In Senator Tomasi's case, we are prepared to treat him with five antibodies carrying three different drugs. This is the first time a multiple warhead arrangement has been prepared. We have Adriamycin, cis-platinum, and Mitomycin C all loaded on the antibody cocktail. I'd like to show a series of slides so you can see the impact this approach has on treating the Senator's tumor in mice."

Dr. Belner flashed up on the screen a slide showing a sickly looking tiny mouse without any hair, with a big, bulging tumor on its side.

"This is the nude mouse before treatment with the cocktail, no warhead."

Next slide. The mouse looked even sicklier, the tumor even larger.

"As you can see, the antibody cocktail without the attached drugs had no effect."

Next slide; another mouse; another huge tumor.

"This is Senator Tomasi's lymphoma growing in a mouse, before treatment with an antibody-Adriamycin single drug conjugate."

In the next slide the tumor was obviously reduced, but still present. The mouse didn't look too happy.

"So, you can see that the Adriamycin worked, and the tumor is reduced, although not gone. Now, we pulled some cells out of what's left of that tumor, grew them in another mouse, and treated it again with the Adriamycin conjugate." Another slide, a mouse with a large tumor.

"As you can see, these residual cells were resident to Adriamycin. Therefore, Senator Tomasi's lymphoma has several clones of cells. All express the proteins that provide antibody formation, but some of the cells are resistant to Adriamycin. So we feel that multiple drug delivery is the way to go, just as multiple drug chemotherapy has been more effective than single drugs in treating lymphoma. Thus, we've prepared this cocktail of five antibody hooked to three drugs, and I want to show you these effects in the mouse."

This time a slide flashed on the screen with five nude mice laid out adjacent to one another, tumors bulging from their hairless sides.

"As you can see, we have Senator Tomasi's lymphoma cells growing in the flasks of these mice. All have advanced tumors and all are systemically ill. All were treated with the five antibody cocktail hooked to the three drugs."

The next slide came up. The mice were again held down and laid out, but no tumors were visible. "Now, here are these mice three months later." All five were up in the cage looking perfectly healthy. "We have followed these animals for more than six months, and none have had a recurrence of the tumor." Dr. Belner looked around at the excited expressions on his colleagues' faces.

"This is the most striking experiment we've ever done at CTI. It is the most rewarding experiment I've been associated with in over ten years in the laboratory. I must tell you that I'm having trouble stifling my enthusiasm. I can't guarantee that Senator Tomasi will react as these mice have, but based on our experience with Adriamycin, which did translate rather well from mouse to man, I predict that this multiple warhead approach could be a real breakthrough." Dick Belner sat down. Everyone in the room had heard fragments of the experiments as they were being conducted, but the final presentation was very exciting. First there was silence. Then applause and the room was abuzz.

Robert Gordon stood. "I'd like to be sure you are all putting this in the proper perspective. We've all seen miraculous mouse cures before. But the tumor cells growing in these mice are the same as those in Senator Tomasi, nothing artificial. Indeed, we've grown his tumor cells from before chemotherapy as well as after, and this clone of resistant cells has clearly arisen since Adriamycin chemotherapy put him into remission. I think we have defined most of the tumor cell biology of the Senator's multiclonal lymphoma."

"I've called you all here today because I spoke earlier with the Senator. He has noticed a new lymph node swelling in his neck. I think the time has come to do the experiment, and he agrees. It's time, as we say in the South, to fish or cut bait. To deploy our first multiple warhead immunoconjugate in a man, not a mouse. He'll be down here for treatment next week. Dick, do we have sufficient amounts of antibody cocktail prepared and ready?"

Dr. Belner nearly jumped out of his seat. "Yes, yes. We have eight grams of antibody. Loaded onto those eight grams is nearly one gram of Adriamycin, nearly two grams of cis-platinum, and more than 500 milligrams of Mito C."

"Great! Given as chemotherapy, that's probably ten times the lethal dose. Now we'll see what happens. He's had a lot of chemotherapy, so his bone marrow will be quite sensitive," Dr. Gordon said. "If these drugs are properly directed away from normal tissues and into the tumor, he could have a good clinical response with no severe suppression of his blood counts. If we're wrong, and the drugs are not well-directed, not only will the experiment fail, but the Senator will as well."

"If this works, can we title the paper 'The Making of a President'?" quipped Belner.

CHAPTER 26

FULL CIRCLE

Fall 1986

The rumor mill was running hot and heavy at the FCI. The press was in a feeding frenzy, not knowing which story to concentrate on -- the mysterious personal life of Stanley Lizzard, or the exposed managerial shenanigans of Stephen Musso. The FCI was at the same time virtually paralyzed over the Musso investigation, and titillated and distraught over the Lizzard affair. Never before had the Federal Cancer Program been rocked by such scandal.

The problem with Stanley Lizzard was of a highly personal nature. His fever, enlarged lymph nodes, sweats, rash and most recently purplish skin sores meant only one thing. Stanley had denied it for awhile, but repeated examinations, tests and biopsies proved it beyond any doubt - - he had AIDS. It was a personal tragedy, and a source of unwanted publicity for the FCI. Stephen himself had interceded and tried to keep things as quiet as possible but was unsuccessful. Besides, he had his own troubles. Poor Stanley looked terrible and hadn't been seen in his office for weeks. He was now said to be under treatment in a private Bethesda hospital. And of course, the press was everywhere.

Rumors about Stanley abounded: He was a closet homosexual; he had had sexual relations with a prostitute and intravenous drug user from 14th Street who was later found to be infected by the AIDS virus; a disgruntled laboratory worker had spiked the virus into Stanley's coffee after she was discharged for starting rumors about cell contamination and the spiking of cultures with viruses in Roger Salla and George

Trumpey's laboratories. It seemed that each day brought a new tale.

But the attention being given Stanley's misfortune would soon die down, Stephen knew, as soon as something more tantalizing arose.

The big news was the investigation. Unlike Stanley's battle with AIDS, the FCI investigation had long term implications which could impact on the Federal Cancer Program and the $1.5 billion handed out each year.

The focus of the scandal was a series of articles written for the Washington Post by post-doc turned reporter Martin Bartholomew. The first article, which appeared on July 4, 1986, had hit the town like a bombshell. The topic was peer review, with Bartholomew citing twelve specific instances in which committees had been intentionally set up to achieve a certain end. The best characterized was the review of Dr. George Trumpey and his laboratory. The other examples were less spectacular, less obvious, but they added up to quite a story. Another interesting case was the odd grant review for Dr. Cliner. A multi-staged review and appeal process, quite unusual in depth and scope, appeared to have taken place. A relationship to Senator Haller, a senior senator from Utah who directed an earlier FCI expose was postulated.

In every instance, Stephen Musso or one of his close associates had played a major role in the selection of the peer review committee, and the results achieved seemed to be consistent with a pattern of stated goals or private statements on the part of Dr. Musso prior to the review.

Martin Bartholomew was a man of several talents. His inside knowledge of both the science and politics at the FCI, combined with his ability to craft a compelling article, seriously threatened the usually unflappable Stephen Musso. Bartholomew's engagement to a Ms. Constance Kelly received brief mention in the Post. A Florida marriage was planned for September. The Washington Post series was beautifully chronicled, with more than adequate supporting data. Like all newspaper articles, there was some conjecture and room for doubt, but it was obvious to everyone that Bartholomew had done his homework.

The second bombshell dropped just a week after the first, when Stephen was still reeling from the realization that the dangerous post-doc Bartholomew could have gotten his hands on some truly damaging evidence. All it took was a sharp mind to put it all together and it looked like he had just that sort of mind. The second piece dealt with the chemotherapy development program. This report was less specific than the first but its scope was enormous. It traced a ten year story of resource allocation that appeared to show striking favoritism for the view that chemicals, randomly identified from among the millions of compounds in the environment, might include substances with strong anticancer activity. To date, literally millions of chemicals had been screened, either by analysis or by computer modeling, and from these a series of drugs had been developed showing anticancer activity.

There was nothing wrong with screening the environment for cancer-killing compounds. But what was suspicious was that so many of the accepted chemicals were strikingly similar, attacking the cancer cells with similar mechanisms. And all were highly toxic. Even more curious was in spite of the broadly held view that anticancer drug development in the pharmaceutical industry had hit a plateau, and in contrast to much of the scientific community which had suggested that the approach was becoming increasingly less productive, FCI had actually increased spending for drugs over the last five years. It didn't make sense. Except, as Martin carefully chronicled, the money kept going to the same "old boys," friends and family of Stephen Musso. The same scientists, the same clinicians, the same "pipeline" university programs. The explanation that these were simply the best scientists who repeatedly received funds and new drugs was met with considerable skepticism.

In addition, explanations from FCI officials in response to Congressional requests for information were noted to involve several years of slanting of figures with interpretations that weren't completely factual. Often, when the Institute's support of biological approaches was questioned, the numbers were inflated, including figures from grants that were only peripherally involved or not directly part of the biotherapy program. The numbers went the other way for drug development. The figures were often minimized, categorizing research as basic or not involved in the actual drug development process in an apparent effort to make the level of resources allocated to drugs more consistent with industrial and academic recommendations. Congress was not happy. Investigative committees were being formulated to ferret out the "truth."

Bartholomew summarized the drug development data over the past 15 years and demonstrated, at least by inference, strong selective pressures on the part of FCI management to fund drug development and certain people/institutions to the exclusion of many other promising areas in cancer research and developmental therapeutics. The figures spoke for themselves -- Bartholomew didn't even need to prove that the process of advice and consent provided by peer review to drive the allocation of FCI resources was being completely subverted. This was obvious to all who read the report. Musso and his associates were cited as the controlling force behind those misallocations.

The third and final article was more personal but no less damaging. Over the past 15 years, a series of scientists and clinicians had worked at the FCI, each making important discoveries along the way. They had worked long and hard on creative, pet projects, only to see their laboratory chief or collaborator become the first author, taking credit for the work. Anyone who dared to protest was quickly silenced, labelled a malcontent, found to be less effective over time with a personnel folder that precisely reflected the low productivity and soon afterwards "voluntarily" left for an opportunity outside of government that was simply too good to turn down. Others were out in the street with a sudden lack of opportunity in research.

The final article was surgical and precise. Every major event that Stephen had engineered since 1980 was identified. It was as if this investigator had lived with Musso and had access to all of his personal notes and records. Or had heard the verbal interactions or had been intimate with him. Bartholomew had dug deeply into FCI records for documentation, and now reported on individuals whose personnel evaluations had changed dramatically from one review period to the next. These downswings predictably occurred shortly before the individual's often hasty resignation. An event and a researcher's role in it would appear one way at the time it happened, but the story was recorded another way in his file six months or a year later. It was as if history was being rewritten. Over and over again, a highly productive, well respected scientist would suddenly be painted as a virtual idiot. The transitions illustrated by Bartholomew were riveting.

And he took it one step further, following the ill-fated investigators' careers after they left the FCI. Typically, a researcher would become associated with some respected institution, and since he was still involved in cancer research, would write grants to the FCI for funding. But they seldom passed peer review. His funding would gradually diminish and he would ultimately disappear as a leader. There were a handful of exceptions, people who went to pharmaceutical companies or privately funded ventures, those who continued to do the high-quality work they had always done, in spite of the federal process. But for most, their careers were forever ruined, sometimes with tragic personal consequences.

The one thing that all of these uprooted researchers had in common was a run-in with Stephen Musso.

The Washington Post three-part series was only the tip of the iceberg of unknown proportions. Martin Bartholomew had spent more than four years on the investigation -- one year in thinking about it, two years of working for the FCI and one year of writing and preparing. Connie's hand in the work was apparent to Stephen. Much of the information had to result from this guy's knowing which file to search. Someone had to have access to personnel files, memoranda and official files in a manner far beyond the post-doc Bartholomew. Someone had to help who knew where the bodies were buried. But why, why had Connie done this? It was obvious that they had a larger goal in mind. What did they want? His job? A book? A movie?

The Washington Post series merely whetted the appetite of the East Coast audience. And as the articles were picked up by newspapers and magazines throughout the country, the impact of the scandal become more intense. Donahue and Oprah Winfrey wanted Martin on their shows. Bartholomew was already halfway through a book being written for a leading New York publishing house. And on the West Coast there was talk of the inevitable screenplay. What a story!

And what a wonderful movie it would make! An agency set up for the public good, with goals beyond reproach. Cancer research with taxpayer dollars. Mother and apple pie. Yet within the hallowed system were rotten apples, individuals who used public money and the system to their own personal benefit, turning the publicly-funded FCI into a kingdom run by one man, Stephen Musso. It was the story of a mafia family.

Martin Bartholomew's hard work had paid off. He was granting interviews, discussing his methods, and all the while disseminating the story of corruption. Washington was abuzz, and Congress was hot.

"Dr. Musso, did you play any role in selecting the committee that reviewed Dr. George Trumpey's laboratory in 1982?"

"Absolutely not, that process is on automatic pilot at the cancer institute. Committee members are chosen from lists of qualified individuals and program directors simply go down the list and select people to fill the committee needs. From time to time, I have exerted some influence on the selection of a chairman, but only when I felt that a particular person brought a special expertise to the review process. But over and above that, these were simply standard peer review processes," Dr. Musso answered.

The Senator droned on, question after question. And the answers were consistently well structured, well thought out, and plausible.

In dollar terms this FCI business was actually pretty small potatoes for the Senate Committee. They had looked into mismanagement and fraud by the Pentagon, difficulties in the Justice Department, and contract misappropriations by the Department of Commerce. By their standards, the amounts being talked about at the FCI were not all that great, and there was little suggestion of personal financial benefit, a major focus of their inquiry. But something was going on, and they would spend a few days illustrating their interest to the American public. Cancer was important. Congress didn't like being deceived. The media was interested and votes would result.

Dr. Musso proved to be a superb witness. His staff had prepared him well, supplying every minute detail. So he had an eloquent and plausible answer to every query, a perfectly logical explanation for every allegation. He was always scientific, reasonable, and always appearing to work in the public interest. He was a man with a great deal of credibility in Congress. He was a consummate politician; a fine actor.

But behind the scenes, the Washington Post series had done irreversible damage. And now Stephen was beginning to get a taste of his own medicine. He was asked to attend a private meeting of the President's Cancer Panel, the august body of three that watched over the Federal Cancer Advisory Board and the Federal Cancer Institute. Their conclusion was firm. Stephen Musso had become a liability for the administration. While the right and wrong of his actions could be debated back and forth, the public impact was clear. He was hurting the

President, focusing attention on problems in the administration. There were enough such problems in Washington and the President wanted a quick fix on this one.

It was time for Stephen to move on.

CHAPTER 27

THE PRIZE

1987

Roger Salla's instincts had been correct. The lymphoma virus announcement had indeed stirred a great deal of attention and the power hungry Stephen had directly profited from it -- a second Wilson prize, media attention, praise from his colleagues. But despite these career boosts, the big prize for 1985 had passed him by.

Roger couldn't help but smile at how marvelously things were going for him. Stephen's recent problem had directed attention away from his clinical and scientific accomplishments, but it had virtually no impact on Roger's work. Best of all, Bartholomew's didn't include Roger in his reports on FCI mischief. The support pipeline that Stephen had so carefully put into place for Roger continued to deliver running on auto pilot even as the head man was being publicly exposed. In Roger's laboratory, the money continued to flow, the facilities operated efficiently, and Roger's strategy of waiting to announce the colon cancer virus was successful beyond his wildest dreams.

Charlie Templeton's work was right on target. There was indeed a virus in the colon cancer cells, and the fermentation plant at Arlington relieved of its previous biotherapy chores, had produced gram quantities, pounds really, of cells for analysis. The virus was present in miniscule amounts, difficult to see, almost impossible to detect, but nonetheless present, lurking as an integral part of the cellular metabolic machinery. Roger's team was not only able to prove the existence of the virus, but to isolate it and grow it in other tissue culture cells.

The process was complete, totally erasing his human leukemia virus mistake of so long ago. The lymphoma discovery was a step in the right direction, but the colon cancer virus was big news, a stunning finishing touch.

Roger carefully orchestrated reports on his findings in a way to maximize their impact. He reported in Journal of Science on the antibodies against the virus they had found in colon cancer patients which confirmed the virus' existence in patients. A simultaneous article in Natural Science outlined the process of virus isolation and propogation, with the definitive proof that the virus was in fact a cause of colon cancer. And finally, a preliminary clinical trial report in the Journal of Clinical Medicine on the use of a human aantibody made in Roger's laboratory as therapy for patients with advanced colon cancer. He put Templeton's name only on the Nature article. With Roger as the senior author on all three papers, he was obviously the "discoverer" of the new virus. This strategy of being the only common author on a series of related papers always worked.

Taken together, these three classic papers established formal proof that, at least for some patients with colon cancer, a virus was associated and was probably the causative agent. Since antibody could be generated to that virus that might be useful in treatment the medical community saw this as a major therapeutic discovery, not just a sterile piece of science in tumor biology. Roger was pleased. Like Stephen Musso, he had come full circle and everything was to hit the press this week.

Stockholm

It was the year's biggest celebration. The gigantic banquet hall was packed with thousands of penguin-like men and decked-out women, each trying to be noticed, if not for their beauty, at least for their costume. It was the yearly Nobel Prize ceremony. At the formal head table sat selected Nobel laureates. As always, the King and Queen were in attendance.

All was silent as the chairman of the committee that had made the selections for the Nobel prizes in physiology and medicine ascended the podium. Everyone knew who was to win the prize this year. Dr. Roger Salla had carefully orchestrated his announcements through major journals, and there was no questions that his discovery of a virus for colon cancer was the most important stride forward in cancer research in more than two decades. In fact, a putative colon cancer virus had been sought for over 40 years. The discovery had led to discussion of whether this was the sole cause or if it worked with a co-factor, and there was much talk about possible therapeutic implications. Now, all of Roger Salla's work seemed to flow together as a carefully planned research tour de force, first the HV-A and B series, then HLV-1, and now the colon cancer virus, CCV 1. Dr. Salla and the FCI group at his command led the world in isolating and characterizing viruses associated with human malignancies.

In the glory surrounding Roger Salla's Prize, Charlie Templeton was all but forgotten, absorbed into the all-encompassing group of "others" behind the one great mind. Such was the way of big science.

"Ladies and gentlemen, it is my great pleasure to announce the 1987 Nobel Prize for Medicine or Physiology to go to the discoverer of the virus that is an important cause if not the sole cause of the most common human malignancy in the United States and a major health problem throughout the world, colon cancer. Never before has a Nobel been given within one year of a discovery. Such is the importance of this discovery. This man, through the dedicated efforts of literally hundreds of scientists and thousands of technicians stretching over more than a decade has relentlessly tracked this virus and several others as a cause of human cancer. May I present to each of you Dr. Roger Salla, Nobel Laureate in medicine 1987."

A great standing ovation followed, one which seemed to surpass the usual recognition in a Nobel ceremony. Perhaps it was because this discovery promised to have direct treatment implications in the short term, or perhaps it was more personal, the fact that everyone present knew someone with cancer.

As he stepped to the podium, Roger could sense a kaleidoscope of his life passing before him. Years of 18 hour-a-day, seven-days-a-week work, driving a team toward the ultimate accomplishment. He thought fleetingly of Charlie Templeton, who had made the original observations, but of course it was his guidance and resources that had transformed Templeton's hypotheses into reality. Briefly, guilt touched his forebrain. All the people he had used over the years. But only briefly. Salla had received other honors -- the De Vincio Medal, the Lister Scroll, the Wilson Prize, but all paled in comparison to this unforgettable moment, this unforgettable Prize. He had attained his life dream.

Roger Salla was living proof that the system worked. An enormous expenditure of funds by a single government agency, given to a single talented scientist, could result in major discoveries. There were those who despised Roger Salla, and there were many who questioned his motives, but no one could argue with the simple fact that more money, more scientists, more laboratories, and more effort could accomplish almost any reasonable scientific goal. Big science worked. Roger proved it again.

Stephen Musso and the scientists whose careers he had ruined were gone, Sam Fish and the other henchmen forgotten, Stanley Lizzard dead. But the Roger Sallas and the system would live and grow and continue to work. Privatization may indeed find a niche, but it paled next to the power of the government, the power of Big Science. Massive public subsidy, no risk of litigation, non-profit, public service, mother and apple pie, and the support of federal bureaucracy were tools of undeniable magnitude in the conduct of research.

And the crowd worshipped.

EPILOGUE

DANIEL WEIL

Daniel Weil responded to the careful administration of Interleukin-2/activated cells by CTI. Although the tumor mass shrunk to a barely detectable size on the plain chest X-ray, his CT scan continued to show persistent disease. The remission lasted four months, at which time he was retreated with the same approach, this time with no effect. Chemotherapy, which hadn't worked earlier, was administered again, and this time he had a response. It lasted another six months.

In spite of further chemotherapy and biotherapy, Daniel Weil died quietly at his home in Groton, Connecticut on December 4, 1987 at the age of 86. He fought a gallant, personal battle and remained optimistic to the end. His battle of some seven years with lung cancer was much longer than the average four to six months for most patients with this disease. He illustrated how power and influence could be currencies in the government system. Access through influence. Although standard as well as experimental treatment ultimately failed, Mr. Weil was testimony to the positive effects of an aggressive, individualized approach to cancer treatment using the research laboratory. He was a pioneer in validating the private alternative in research based cancer treatment.

JOHN J. OWENS

John J. Owens received massive doses of a mouse monoclonal antibody cocktail hooked to Mitomycin C, administered through his intrahepatic arterial catheter, his "second bellybutton." The cocktail consisted of three types of antibodies, each loaded with nearly 40 molecules of drug. Complete regression of his liver metastasis occurred, and no further evidence of disease developed for the ensuing six months. John J. was re-explored at Good Samaritan Hospital on September 16, 1987, and no evidence of cancer could be found in his liver. His "button" was removed, and he continues in complete remission. His "Task Force" was disbanded but John J. is CTIs and Robert Gordon's most ardent supporter. He continues to invest in cancer research and pump millions of dollars yearly into a fund for patients, medically eligible but not financially able to pursue CTIs services.

SAM LURIA

Sam Luria continued to enjoy life with stable disease through 1987. The three universities which held the hybridomas making antibodies that reacted with his myeloma cells deliberated for another eight months, then decided not to make the hybridomas available for his treatment. Their stance was that CTI was commercializing antibodies prematurely. Sam Luria, private citizen, was denied access to their taxpayer-generated antibodies. On October 4, 1987, Sam filed suite in Federal Court asking that these publicly funded universities release the antibodies in question. That suit is pending.

He was brought to Good Samaritan Hospital and large quantities of bone marrow were removed under general anesthesia. The myeloma cells were separated from his normal bone marrow elements and mice were immunized with them. CTI is currently screening and selecting antibodies that might be useful in his future treatment. Fortunately, Sam Luria's disease has not progressed significantly and he appears to have time to wait for the research project to go to completion. Sam is currently on the telephone organizing a political action group to look into public funded research and the limited availability through the government/university system of cells, antibodies and other biologicals for patient treatment.

LYDIA GREEN

Lydia Green was treated with an antibody cocktail hooked to Adriamycin. She had become resistant to multiple forms of chemotherapy and exhibited very poor bone marrow tolerance to further drug treatment. Biotherapy was the only avenue for her.

She tolerated the antibody-Adriamycin conjugates very well with minimal toxicity and went into complete remission. All evidence of lymph node enlargement and chest fluid disappeared. However, five months later a new lymph node appeared in the left neck, and biopsy revealed the cells to be resistant to Adriamycin. She had developed an allergy to the mouse protein and couldn't be retreated with the same antibodies. Research was begun to attempt to develop human antibodies that could be used in subsequent treatment. Unfortunately, she developed massive intercranial bleeding and died on July 4, 1987. Postmortem revealed multiple areas of lymphoma with all of the cells resistant to Adriamycin. Cause of death was a ruptured blood vessel in the brain unrelated to her lymphoma.

SENATOR TOMASI

Senator Tomasi was the first person in the world to be treated with a custom-tailored cocktail of five antibodies conjugated to three drugs. After treatment, he went into complete remission and is currently without any evidence of active lymphoma. Because sensitive assays are available to measure idiotype levels as a marker for the Senator's lymphoma, Dr. Gordon was able to assure Tomasi and his political constituency that the lymphoma was gone. The Senator was cured. He feels quite well. Plans are underway to recapture the Senate seat in 1990, and his constituents are making preliminary plans for the Presidency in 1992. His bout with cancer, and his victory, seem to have won him broad public support. He found "the cure" and can now return to changing the political system.

STANLEY LIZZARD

The source of the HIV-1 was never documented or disclosed. Dr. Lizzard's AIDS became complicated by the skin nodules of Kaposi's sarcoma. In spite of aggressive treatment with interferon, Interleukin-2/activated cells, AZT and chemotherapy, he succumbed to massive lung infection with pneumocystis carinii pneumonia in Bethesda General Hospital November 12, 1986.

ROGER SALLA

Dr. Salla received the Nobel Prize in physiology and medicine in 1987, and worldwide acclaim continues, although subsequent trials of antibody to the colon cancer virus proved ineffectual. Antiviral drugs were equally unrewarding. Most scientists now believe that the colon virus, though causative, plays little role in the disease after apparent cancer is present in the patient. Research efforts are now underway to characterize the cell surface molecules induced by the virus in an attempt to develop a possible vaccine. On another front, Salla's research team, with Charlie Templeton now second in command, is presently investigating breast cancer as another common human malignancy that might harbor a virus.

STEPHEN MUSSO

On July 15, 1987, after nearly a year of investigation and controversy, Stephen Musso resigned as Director of the FCI. The official press release from Cancer Communications read:

> *"It is with great pride that I leave the Federal Cancer Institute. My work has been possible because of the support of the public, the support of my fellow researchers, and the long term support of my patients. I am pleased with the Institute's record of accomplishment during my tenure as Director and as I leave the government, I believe the Institute will continue in its leadership position as the flagship of cancer research for the world.*
>
> *It is with great anticipation that I return to New York, the city of my original training, to take on the scientific directorship of BMA Pharmaceutical Company. BMA has long been a world class pharmaceutical leader with first class programs in drug development. BMA's track record of eight anticancer drugs approved for clinical use in five years is a great achievement, unmatched in the industry. I believe with my expertise, BMA can do even more."*

He didn't mention the $950,000 yearly salary, the stock option arrangement, his recent divorce, or his soon to be consummated marriage toMelody Murman.

He was eloquent to the very end.

MARTIN BARTHOLOMEW

After the Washington Post series, Martin was called to testify before three Senate committees. This publicity helped make his book, "The Cancer Institute Family," a bestseller. The movie, title to be determined, will premiere in the summer of

1990. He and wife, Connie, currently live in Beverly Hills, California.

ROBERT GORDON

Dr. Robert Gordon lives and works in Fairfield, Georgia. His company, Cancer Therapeutics Inc., continues to prosper. After its public offering, sufficient resources were in place to expand the operation and by the end of 1987, plans were underway to establish six regional laboratories around the United States and four around the world. There continues to be a major interest on the part of the media, patients, and physicians in this private approach that so directly links patients to cancer research and treatment.